the analytic situation

How Patient and Therapist Communicate

the analytic situation

How Patient and Therapist Communicate

Edited by Hendrik M. Ruitenbeek

Routledge
Taylor & Francis Group
LONDON AND NEW YORK

First published 1973 by Transaction Publishers

2 Park Square, Milton Park, Abingdon, Oxfordshire OX14 4RN
711 Third Avenue, New York, NY 10017

Routledge is an imprint of the Taylor & Francis Group, an informa business

First issued in hardback 2017

Library of Congress Catalog Number: 2007026387

Library of Congress Cataloging-in-Publication Data

Ruitenbeek, Hendrik Marinus, 1928-
The analytic situation : how patient and therapist communicate / Hendrik M. Ruitenbeek.
p. ; cm.
Originally published: Chicago : Aldine, c1973.
Includes bibliographical references and index.
ISBN 978-0-202-30987-3 (alk. paper)
1. Psychoanalysis. 2. Psychotherapist and patient. I. Title.
[DNLM: 1. Psychotherapeutic Processes--Collected Works. 2. Psychoanalytic Therapy--methods--Collected Works. WM 420 R933a 2007]

RC480.5.R83 2007
616.89'17--dc22

2007026387

ISBN 13: 978-0-202-30987-3 (pbk)
ISBN 13: 978-1-138-53426-1 (hbk)

Contents

Introduction

Psychoanalysis is changing in our contemporary society. The days are long past when psychoanalysis and psychoanalytic thinking were the cherished property of a knowledgeable few, the "Viennese intimi," and the following period where psychoanalysis was practiced primarily by the successors to the early Vienna circle. Although depth analysis is still very much the privilege of the educated and often sophisticated urban middle class, radical changes have occurred in the psychoanalytic situation.

More and more we have come to realize that psychoanalysis in its early years was a rather informal affair. The pioneer analysts—for example, Ferenczi and Rank—were rather active and informal with their patients. Some of them even had not been analyzed themselves, Abraham for example, and the psychoanalytic practice in that time was more of an adventurous affair than it is today. The relationship between analysts and patients was certainly different. Analysts had not yet examined their counter-transference reactions and often got themselves involved in the personal lives of their patients and *vice versa*. They moved in the same social circle and often they knew each other's friends. This colored the analytic experience of that time. The rules and regulations were a part of the second-generation analysts, who as a result became far more rigid and uptight than they should have been.

Not only have new thinkers in psychotherapy—the Gestaltists, the Existentialists, the neo-Freudians, the Behaviorists, the members of the rational-emotive school, the ego-psychologists, the proponents of encounter groups, and many others—presented us with extreme departures from what was termed orthodox therapy, but many conventional and orthodox therapists have questioned and reviewed the various dynamics of the psychoanalytic situation itself. They realized that their patients had changed from the type who were seen in Vienna in 1910 and noticed also that they themselves were sometimes quite flexible in experimenting within the psychoanalytic situation.

Masud Khan, in what amounts to a plea for tolerance among analysts concerning one's own techniques and approaches to the analytic situation, remarks:

> We analysts seem to have a poor tolerance of each other's style and sensibility of clinical handling of the patient. We tend to hide or understate the truly personal creative ventures in our clinical work, because we fear that to seek help through a candid discussion would provoke only envy or carping criticism from our colleagues. Hence our theory of the standard analytic technique poorly reflects the richness of the actual tradition of clinical work as it has evolved over the past four decades.[1]

The Freudian psychoanalyst, Ralph Greenson, pleads for the role of psychoanalyst as innovator in the psychoanalytic situation. "The innovator psychoanalyst is an adventurer, a risk-taker, an explorer. His curiosity leads him to investigate the unknown. This may indicate a freedom from anxiety or a counterphobic attitude. In any event, the anxiety is overridden by the urge to know, to explore. Innovators are not awed by tradition, nor are they lovers of conformity. They are willing to risk being wrong and to expose themselves to the attacks of their colleagues."[2]

The intimate interaction between analyst and patient is full of possibilities and hazards. As Freud warned:

> The principal battle in psychoanalysis is that of transference. . . . This struggle between the doctor and the patient, between intellect and instinctual life, between understanding and seeking to act, is played out almost exclusively in the phenomena of transference. It is on that field that the victory must be won—the victory whose expression is the permanent cure of the neurosis.[3]

As psychoanalysis has grown, analysts of every school have come to realize the importance of Freud's statement on transference in the analytic situation. One could almost paraphrase Freud's classic statement on the id in the following words: "Where there is no transference, there is no analysis." The paper included here on transference is by Melanie Klein, who became one of England's most outstanding

1. M. Masud R. Khan, "On Symbiotic Omnipotence," *The Psychoanalytic Forum*, Vol. III, 1969, p. 158.
2. Ralph R. Greenson, "The Origin and Fate of New Ideas in Psychoanalysis," *International Journal of Psycho-Analysis*, Vol. 50, Part 4, 1969, p. 509.
3. Sigmund Freud, "The Dynamics of Transference," *Standard Edition*, Vol.

analysts in the 1930s. She was very close to the first generation of analysts and was one of the first students at the Berlin Psychoanalytic Institute at a time when this institute was still rather small and informal. Her impact on British psychoanalysis has been substantial, albeit highly controversial. Although she acquired an enormous reputation in the field of child psychoanalysis, her influence and place in British psychoanalysis is tied to her thesis on the pre-oedipal stage, which shook the British psychoanalytic society to its very foundations. In her paper on transference she develops the notion that we deal not only with positive transference in our relationship with patients, but to an even greater extent with negative transference, a subject still very difficult to handle for many analysts, especially the younger analysts. Although the paper was written some time ago it has lost none of its freshness and originality of thought.

Even well-trained, experienced, and well-analyzed therapists are often at a loss when faced with certain unexpected events in the psychoanalytic situation. The literature of psychoanalysis offers much material on psychoanalytic techniques and on dreams and fantasies, but tells little about the specific encounters that may face analysts and patients in their mutual relationship.

Questions such as silence, laughter, crying, the role of touch, and the role of gifts in therapy have often been considered somewhat annoying or even embarrassing to both the therapist and the patient. Much of the difficulty, as might be expected, is connected with the flexibility of the analyst in the therapeutic situation. Flexibility and tranquility have never been among the major assets of the contemporary therapist. The casual attitude of some of the pioneer therapists disappeared rather quickly as psychoanalysis became increasingly formalized. In the account of her personal analysis with Sachs, Bryher emphasizes the easy attitude toward their patients of the early psychoanalysts, including Freud himself, "I was one of the early group of analysands and it was much less stiff (stuffy, I think, would be a more correct word) than it is today."[4] Many other accounts by former patients of the pioneer analysts confirm their informal and relaxed attitude toward their patients.

The formalization and institutionalization of psychoanalysis was probably necessary to assure the status of psychoanalysis, and certain ground rules and regulations had to be laid down, but they took away the kind of informal attitude toward patients that existed in

---

XII (London: Hogarth, 1958), p. 108.

4. Bryher, *The Heart to Artemis* (New York: Harcourt, Brace & World, 1962), pp. 253-254.

the early days of psychoanalysis. As soon as psychoanalysis lost its early experimental aspects and subsequently gained in respectability, it unfortunately acquired some of the rigid aspects of what we now call orthodox or "Freudian" psychoanalysis.

And so psychoanalysis arrived at a stage in which experimentation was discouraged, and a great deal of the spontaneity and inventive spirit of early psychoanalysis disappeared during the "adolescence" of psychoanalysis. Followers of Freud, especially the second generation of psychoanalysts, became rigid and inflexible in their psychoanalytic practice and theory. Dissenters were dismissed during Freud's life, and the psychoanalytic establishment began to be stricter in the practice of psychoanalysis than Freud himself. Indeed, it seems that Freud's pupils and close associates were more eager to eliminate the dissenters than Freud was. Certainly, people who have recorded their memories of being analyzed by Freud testify to his liberal mind and tolerant attitude in therapy.[5] Everything I have read by or about Freud convinces me that he would have been distressed at the closed mindedness of many of his followers.

This rigidity was not conducive to discussion of the various difficulties, the often delicate problems that arose in the psychoanalytic situation. In the absence of serious consideration of the issues of the therapeutic situation, the way was opened for "wild" experimentation,[6] sometimes inadequately thought through, sometimes dangerously exploitive. Because orthodox analysts frequently ignored the problem, patient-therapist relationships often were left to the "crackpots" by default.

Only in the last decade or so have more conventional psychoanalysts started to discuss some of the questions raised by therapists of new schools of thought. More Freudian analysts have become convinced that their commitment to psychotherapy and to the therapeutic situation implies a need to keep mind and eye open to new developments in psychotherapy. They, too, are gradually shifting their role from distant listener and interpreter to fellow human being personally involved with the patient in the therapeutic situation.

Because contemporary patients differ considerably from the people Freud and his early pupils treated, they are less inclined to

5. Some of these recollections are collected in my book, *Freud: As We Knew Him* (Detroit: Wayne University Press, 1973).

6. See S. Freud, " 'Wild' Psychoanalysis," *Standard Edition*, Vol. XI, p. 219. Georg Groddeck delivered a paper on "wild" psychoanalysis at The Congress of the International Psychoanalytic Association on Sept. 9, 1920. It was never published. For further reference see Carl M. Grossman and Sylvia Grossman, The Wild Analyst (New York: George Braziller, 1965).

accept the burdens of the past and are more concerned about their situation in the present. They are more alert to the psychoanalytic process *per se* because they are far better acquainted with psychoanalytic ideas. They are more interested in what is happening in the process of analysis.[7]

Analysts have become more daring, too, and the "Why" so often directed to the patient, has become "Why not."[8] It is clear that the members of the American Psychoanalytic Association are not the only therapists to be considered qualified psychoanalysts. A vast number of psychologists and social psychologists (and a substantially growing number of capable social workers) have turned to the professional practice of psychotherapy and are often working in the American hinterlands or in low-fee mental health clinics, far from the comfort enjoyed by psychoanalysts in New York or Beverly Hills.[9] These analysts are part of the community in which they live. Their wives know their patients; their children probably go to school with the children of their patients. Traditional taboos on encounters and social interaction between patient and therapist simply cannot be maintained. Even analysts who practice in large cities where they might never meet a patient outside the consulting room may now need to take a fresh view of their approach to social interaction with patients. Admittedly, some of the newer individual and group therapies have already done much in breaking down some of the artificial barriers between the patient and the therapist. The existential therapists have long advocated a more open and humane attitude of the therapist toward the transference situation, but therapists themselves must work to function comfortably with the patient in the transference situation.

In a changing therapeutic situation where the analyst becomes more open and more personal in the interaction with the patient many issues are presented both to the patient and the analyst. Whereas in the classic psychoanalytic situation the analyst is fairly restricted in his communications with his patient and follows a certain predictable pattern, in the more fluid open therapeutic situation the analyst is more vulnerable but also far more involved.

Ruth Cohn believes that all *correct* therapeutic interventions initiate curative processes that affect the patient's total personality.

> This occurs when the intervening stimulus facilitates the patient's recognition of any significant part of important personal reality that he was pre-

7. John Seeley called this the "socialization" of psychoanalysis.
8. For some observations on this point see Medard Boss, *Psychoanalysis and Daseinsanalysis* (New York: Basic Books, 1963), pp. 248-250.
9. Most issues of *Voices*, the publication of the American Academy of Psychotherapists, reflect many aspects of the experiences of the newer therapists.

viously unaware of or detached from. Such curative processes occur when the patient receives messages that help him to: 1) repair distortions in his perceptual and cognitive world, 2) add emotional content to previously deprived or depleted personality areas, 3) free physical mobility from prior rigidity.[10]

Such psychotherapeutic interventions, however, change the picture of the restrained and quiet psychoanalyst to a far more active and engaged person.

> . . . the therapist's task is to strive towards establishing procedures which aim at meeting up with the patient's optimal receptivity and to recognize how he can best function in the patient's interest . . . My hypothesis is that the patient's innate growth potential responds positively to the recognition of any important factor of his personal reality. Therefore the therapist's acceptance of the patient's reality initiates a fluid curative process.[11]

The question of intervention is raised immediately in the discussion in the three papers on silence in this book. Often young analysts, especially, do not know how to respond to their patients' silence, or if they should respond at all! Sasha Nacht, one of France's most distinguished psychoanalysts, examines the role of silence as contrasted to speech and writes that speech is often a clumsy tool in psychoanalysis. His paper shows that silence can indeed be integrated fully into the psychoanalytic process. In "Silence as Communication," M. Masud R. Khan, training analyst at the British Institute of Psychoanalysis and author of many outstanding papers, describes how he dealt with the role of silence in the treatment of an adolescent and how his subtle role as an involved analyst provided the eventual breakthrough for his silent patient. In his essay, Antonio Ferreira stresses the point that silence should be considered an integral part of the relationship between patient and therapist. Ferreira maintains that silence might be as eloquent as the speech in the psychotherapeutic situation.

If silence is an important means of nonverbal communication, there certainly are many other elements of nonverbal nature that are used to communicate in psychoanalysis. Again, inexperienced young analysts are often baffled by the outburst of crying. C. E. Schorer discusses crying and states that it occurs in the psychoanalytic situation as a potent mode of nonverbal communication. The therapist should be alert enough to determine at once if this is a normal or abnormal response. He recommends various courses of

10. Ruth C. Cohn, "Psychoanalytic or Experiental Group Psychotherapy: A False Dichotomy," *The Psychoanalytic Review,* Vol. 56, No. 3, 1969, pp. 333-345.

11. *Ibid.*, p. 334.

action to the therapist confronted with this situation. Interestingly enough, Schorer also raises the question of what the crying of the patient does to the therapist. The crying might force the therapist to reexamine the total psychotherapeutic relationship especially in terms of his own countertransference.

The patient who falls asleep and the patient who does not want to look at the therapist are not uncommon. There are many opinions of what to do or not to do with the patient who falls asleep either on the couch or in the chair. Should the analyst intervene? Most therapists agree that timing is extremely important in approaching such a patient. The English psychoanalyst, Clifford Scott, is represented here by an insightful essay on the roles of sleep and looking at the therapist during the treatment sessions. He introduces a most interesting hypothesis: The total satisfaction of sleep is waking or the act of waking up. He states that more has been written on the subject of sleep as an instinct activity and not so much on the "aim" of the instinct, and he is convinced that the occurrence of sleep during psychotherapy may well mean dealing with many periods of silence, sleepiness, and sleep before the patient approaches understanding of the primary sleep wish and wake wish. According to Scott, more attention should be paid to the patient's defenses against sleeping and looking.

Although little has been written on the subject of how patient and therapist should address each other in the intimate reaction between them, this question is often raised. Some therapists encourage their patients to address them by their first name, others leave it up to the patient, while most therapists probably prefer not to be called by their first names. Why most classically oriented therapists reject first name address is quite obvious. The position of the more orthodox therapist in the therapeutic situation is one of detachment and a degree of impersonality. Undoubtedly, the newer therapists have encouraged an informal attitude and introduced a more humane element in the therapeutic interaction. In such a situation the use of first names could conceivably be useful.

Melvin Selzer advances some speculations about the role and the feelings of the therapist in using first names. It might be that the therapist feels the need to be superior to his patient. It can also possibly include an avoidance of the therapeutic commitment. He raises questions as to the "friendship" approach by the therapist in using first names, while the danger of encouraging regression in the patient by using his first name is very real.

Should we accept gifts from our patients? Should we interpret the motive behind every gift? Should we accept or refuse them without interpretation? Should we give our patients gifts? In his recent book

Brother Animal, Paul Roazen cites Freud as an example and relates that he made substantial financial gifts to patients and former patients.[12] Others have cited Freud's generosity toward them.[13] If therapists accept their patients' gifts, what is the procedure to be followed? How do we interpret this type of *communication* of our patients?

Helen Stein maintains that gifts that are presented during therapy are a special form of communication and have roots in the unconscious fantasy of the patient. In her essay, Dr. Stein traces the origin of gifts in terms of its roots in language, cultural history, and universal symbolism. She says that gifts in therapy symbolize a communion with the past in the universality, symbolism, and archaism of these gifts. Gifts in therapy then, accepted or not, must be interpreted by the therapist. They often may indicate some of the patient's links to his past.

"Are you taking notes?" is one of the first questions a new patient often asks the analyst. It is now generally assumed that it is bad practice to take notes when the patient is sitting up. In such a situation the emphasis is being placed on the interaction–dialogue–between therapist and patient and any writing would distract the patient and thus hamper the lines of communication. Either the analyst must have a good memory or write some notes after the session is over. I have discovered that young analysts who are still in training do want to take notes, if only to get a full picture of the developing analytic situation.

Therapists who do not take notes during the analytic sessions are accustomed to the question of their patients as why they do not take anything down. They ask, "Are you able to remember what I'm saying?" which, of course, indicates an early anxiety about the ability of the therapist. Ira Miller observes that part of the feeling of comfort of the patient at the thought of the therapist's taking notes stems from a wish that the therapist not see what is going on at the moment. Miller feels strongly that the taking of notes during the analytic sessions will serve the resistance of the patient "by virtue of its isolating and intellectualizing the associations." He emphasizes the point that the analytic situation involves two people and that the analyst might want to remove himself from the interaction of the analytic situation by taking notes.

Patients often enter the office, sit down, and then say, "I have a dream, but I don't think it's important enough," or "I think the dream is too short to relate or to make any sense," or "I already

12. See Paul Roazen, *Brother Animal* (New York: Knopf, 1969), pp. 26-27.

13. See Helen Doolittle's account of her analysis with Freud. *Tribute to Freud*, (New York: Pantheon Books).

know what it means," or "You might be interested in the dream, but I'd rather talk about something else," *ad infinitum*! It is, of course, the task of the therapist to take such statements and explore them in cooperation with the patient. Patients often resist their dream material, and the resistance that is obvious in such remarks has to be explored and worked through. In his article, Sandor Feldman illustrates such significant comments made by patients while relating dreams with pertinent clinical material.

When and how to terminate analysis has always been a delicate question for the therapist. Although the literature on this subject is abundant, opinions differ sharply as to the efficacy of setting a termination date. Analysts believe that setting a date might be an impetus to the analysis, or that it might be extremely useful for the successful termination of the analysis, or that it introduces undue anxiety into a situation that is already difficult both for the patient and the analyst. Sandor Ferenczi once believed in setting a date for termination, but later abandoned this practice. Martin Orens explores in great detail and with pertinent clinical material the usefulness of setting a termination date.

There is vast literature on the significance of the fee for psychoanalytic treatment. Every analyst knows how important is the discussion of the fee at the very beginning of the treatment, and he is also aware that many patients try to use the fee to manipulate the analyst and the analytic situation. Sandor Lorand and William A. Console, however, point out that, in contrast to the availability of literature on the fee, there is little written about the patient who is being seen free of charge. In one of his early papers on technique, Freud asked analysts to set aside two hours a week free of charge for patients who are in need. Lorand and Console cite the various conventional hazards of free treatment. Since the patient does not sacrifice anything, there might not be much impetus for him to commit himself fully to the analytic situation. Others, of course, have confirmed this. Many such patients are lax about keeping their appointments and in being punctual. Lorand and Console also discuss the idea that the transference neurosis may not be successfully dealt in a situation where the patient might shy away from his negative feelings about the analyst because he does not pay his share.

In their analytic session, patients will ask "typical" questions such as "When am I getting better?" and "How much longer?" or "Do you see any improvement?" Bradford Wilson examines some typical questions patients ask their therapists in the course of their treatment. Again, most of such questions are forms of *communication* between patient and therapist and require close and careful examination by the therapist. Wilson describes some of the answers that might be given to the patient and our own reactions to these questions.

Patients in psychotherapy tend to hold on to their past. After all, that is all they have at this point in their life. When faced with the necessity of abandoning that past—to be ready for the here-and-now situation—the patient perhaps should be told that he really should mourn the abandoned past. When there is a refusal to mourn—as Sheldon B. Kopp points out—the patient is reluctant to separate himself from what he regrets not having. The patient can only keep what he really had. The patient has to face the fact that he might find life arbitrary and "yet to take things as they are, to bring to them what you can, and to enjoy them as they stand, because this is it . . . " Kopp's approach is akin to many of the contemporary existential attitudes and notions in psychotherapy, and it emphasizes the importance of the present situation for the patient.

In discussing resistance, Joseph Zimmerman uses the term *blockages in therapy* and implies that this term has a wider scope than simple resistance. He describes how, in the course of the psychotherapeutic process, the patient erects, so to say, various blockages or defenses against the therapist and the analysis itself.

The emotional engagement of the therapist and the patient in the psychotherapeutic situation is replete with implications. Unfortunately, too few therapists consider these implications of their emotional engagement with their patients. They often are too afraid of unresolved countertransference feelings really to cope with this type of situation. Questions as to what is "objective" in the psychotherapeutic situation or how detached (if at all) the analyst should be are often avoided. In "Emotional Engagement of Patient and Analyst," Gregory Zilboorg raises the whole question of the "adjusted analyst." How many analysts really go back to their own therapy (or therapist) each five years as Freud recommended? How many analysts are still disturbed themselves? Zilboorg quotes Frink as an example. Although apparently quite unstable in his own personal life, he proved to be a very good therapist. Zilboorg also addresses himself to the question: Should the analyst suppress his own negative feelings about certain patients or voice his feelings and see what happens?

Existential therapists have been dealing with the therapeutic encounter for a long time. They stress it and see the role of the analyst as participant with the patient in the encounter. Hanna Colm feels, and rightly so, that contemporary analysts should *feel* more towards their patients and should not hide behind an authoritative attitude. The therapeutic relationship cannot be prescribed, and she wonders how such a prescribed therapeutic relationship can heal the patient "who may already suffer from lack of trust in genuine relationship to people?"

The encounter also implies a certain flexibility on the part of the therapist, and Edith Weigert, who writes on the flexibility of the therapist and his psychoanalytic techniques, shows once again, what I have maintained throughout my own writings,[14] that Freud had quite a respect for differences in technical style. Weigert maintains that the unconscious of the analyst is a receiving organ, and the countertransference of the analyst becomes a most important source of information in the analytic process. She rightly quotes Otto Fenichel on technical rules: "The observance of a prescribed ceremonial produces a magical impression and may be misinterpreted by the patient in this sense. We know. . . . .that we can and must be elastic in the application of all technical rules." Fenichel goes even further: "Everything is permissible, if only one knows why."

The commitment to one's patients is an important issue with existential analysts. They talk about creating a climate of intimacy between the analyst and the patient. Carl A. Whitaker raises an important question on this issue. How far and how much are we committed to our patients? How much do we give and how much are we *willing* to give? He points out that commitment is not only a commitment for the present but a commitment for the future. If the therapist is ready for such a commitment his own authenticity is established.

Currently the question of touch in psychotherapy has received a great deal of attention. In both group and individual therapy, various methods of physical touch have been employed. Although probably still very much a taboo in orthodox psychoanalytic circles, the use of touch in the psychotherapeutic situation is recognized as a valid tool. Elizabeth Mintz, in her article, has examined the various aspects of touch in psychotherapy and cites some valuable clinical material. We owe especially the Gestalt therapists (and in particular the late Fritz Perls) a debt for pioneering in this particular area.

The nature and identity of the psychotherapist continues to be a probing issue for many therapists themselves. In the fast moving picture of psychoanalysis in this society, we are confronted with new demands from our patients and the society at large. We are forced to examine some of the conventional attitudes with which we were familiar. In the last essay of this book the existential therapist, James F. T. Bugenthal raises some very penetrating questions as to the conventional attitudes of the contemporary therapist.

14. See my own paper, Chapter 23 in this book.

We could not have possibly have covered all the current issues of the psychoanalytic situation. And we are aware of certain omissions, but the issues presented here are an indication of some current preoccupations of both many analysts and patients.

1

MELANIE KLEIN

The Origins of Transference

In his *Fragment of an Analysis of a Case of Hysteria* Freud defines the transference situation in the following way:

> What are transferences? They are new editions or facsimiles of the tendencies and phantasies which are aroused and made conscious during the progress of the analysis; but they have this peculiarity, which is characteristic for their species, that they replace some earlier person by the person of the physician. To put it another way: a whole series of psychological experiences are revived, not as belonging to the past, but as applying to the physician at the present moment.

In some form or other transference operates throughout life and influences all human relations, but here I am only concerned with the manifestations of transference in psychoanalysis. It is characteristic of psycho-analytic procedure that, as it begins to open up roads into the patient's unconscious, his past (in its conscious and unconscious aspects) is gradually being revived. Thereby his urge to transfer his early experiences, object-relations and emotions, is reinforced and they come to focus on the psycho-analyst; this implies that the patient deals with the conflicts and anxieties which have been reactivated, by making use of the same mechanisms and defences as in earlier situations.

It follows that the deeper we are able to penetrate into the unconscious and the further back we can take the analysis, the greater will be our understanding of the transference. Therefore a

Reprinted from the *International Journal of Psychoanalysis*, 1952, Vol. 33, 433-438.

brief summary of my conclusions about the earliest stages of development is relevant to my topic.

The first form of anxiety is of a persecutory nature. The working of the death instinct within–which according to Freud is directed against the organism–gives rise to the fear of annihilation, and this is the primordial cause of persecutory anxiety. Furthermore, from the beginning of post-natal life (I am not concerned here with pre-natal processes) destructive impulses against the object stir up fear of retaliation. These persecutory feelings from inner sources are intensified by painful external experiences, for, from the earliest days onwards, frustration and discomfort arouse in the infant the feeling that he is being attacked by hostile forces. Therefore the sensations experienced by the infant at birth and the difficulties of adapting himself to entirely new conditions give rise to persecutory anxiety. The comfort and care given after birth, particularly the first feeding experiences, are felt to come from good forces. In speaking of "forces" I am using a rather adult word for what the young infant dimly conceives of as objects, either good or bad. The infant directs his feelings of gratification and love towards the "good" breast, and his destructive impulses and feelings of persecution towards what he feels to be frustrating, i.e. the "bad" breast. At this stage splitting processes are at their height, and love and hatred as well as the good and bad aspects of the breast are largely kept apart from one another. The infant's relative security is based on turning the good object into an ideal one as a protection against the dangerous and persecuting object. These processes–that is to say splitting, denial, omnipotence and idealization–are prevalent during the first three or four months of life (which I termed the "paranoid-schizoid position"). In these ways at a very early stage persecutory anxiety and its corollary, idealization, fundamentally influence object relations.

The primal processes of projection and introjection, being inextricably linked with the infant's emotions and anxieties, initiate object-relations; by projecting, i.e. deflecting libido and aggression on to the mother's breast, the basis for object-relations is established; by introjecting the object, first of all the breast, relations to internal objects come into being. My use of the term "object-relations" is based on my contention that the infant has from the beginning of post-natal life a relation to the mother (although focusing primarily on her breast) which is imbued with the fundamental elements of an object-relation, i.e. love, hatred, phantasies, anxieties, and defences.[1]

1. It is an essential feature of this earliest of all object relations that it is the prototype of a relation between *two* people into which no other object enters.

In my view—as I have explained in detail on other occasions—the introjection of the breast is the beginning of superego formation which extends over years. We have grounds for assuming that from the first feeding experience onwards the infant introjects the breast in its various aspects. The core of the superego is thus the mother's breast, both good and bad. Owing to the simultaneous operation of introjection and projection, relations to external and internal objects interact. The father too, who soon plays a role in the child's life, early on becomes part of the infant's internal world. It is characteristic of the infant's emotional life that there are rapid fluctuations between love and hate; between external and internal situations; between perception of reality and the phantasies relating to it; and, accordingly, an interplay between persecutory anxiety and idealization—both referring to internal and external objects; the idealized object being a corollary of the persecutory, extremely bad one.

The ego's growing capacity for integration and synthesis leads more and more, even during these first few months, to states in which love and hatred, and correspondingly the good and bad aspects of objects, are being synthesized; and this gives rise to the second form of anxiety—depressive anxiety—for the infant's aggressive impulses and desires towards the bad breast (mother) are now felt to be a danger to the good breast (mother) as well. In the second quarter of the first year these emotions are reinforced, because at this stage the infant increasingly perceives and introjects the mother as a person. Depressive anxiety is intensified, for the infant feels he has destroyed or is destroying a whole object by his greed and uncontrollable agression. Moreover, owing to the growing synthesis of his emotions, he now feels that these destructive impulses are directed against a *loved person.* Similar processes operate in relation to the father and other members of the family These anxieties and corresponding defences constitute the "depressive position," which comes to a head about the middle of the first year and whose essence is the anxiety and guilt relating to the destruction and loss of the loved internal and external objects.

It is at this stage, and bound up with the depressive position, that

---

This is of vital importance for later object-relations, though in that exclusive form it possibly does not last longer than a very few months, for the phantasies relating to the father and his penis—phantasies which initiate the early stages of the Oedipus complex—introduce the relation to more than one object. In the analysis of adults and children the patient sometimes comes to experience feelings of blissful happiness through the revival of this early exclusive relation with the mother and her breast. Such experiences often follow the analysis of jealousy and rivalry situations in which a third object, ultimately the father, is involved.

the Oedipus complex sets in. Anxiety and guilt add a powerful impetus towards the beginning of the Oedipus complex. For anxiety and guilt increase the need to externalize (project) bad figures and to internalize (introject) good ones; to attach desires, love, feelings of guilt, and reparative tendencies to some objects, and hate and anxiety to others: to find representatives for internal figures in the external world. It is, however, not only the search for new objects which dominates the infant's needs, but also the drive towards new aims: away from the breast towards the penis, i.e. from oral desires towards genital ones. Many factors contribute to these developments: the forward drive of the libido, the growing integration of the ego, physical and mental skills and progressive adaptation to the external world. These trends are bound up with the process of symbol formation, which enables the infant to transfer not only interest, but also emotions and phantasies, anxiety and guilt, from one object to another.

The processes I have described are linked with another fundamental phenomenon governing mental life. I believe that the pressure exerted by the earliest anxiety situations is one of the factors which bring about the repetition compulsion. I shall return to this hypothesis at a later point.

Some of my conclusions about the earliest stages of infancy are a continuation of Freud's discoveries; on certain points, however, divergencies have arisen, one of which is very relevant to my present topic. I am referring to my contention that object-relations are operative from the beginning of post-natal life.

For many years I have held the view that auto-erotism and narcissism are in the young infant contemporaneous with the first relation to objects—external and internalized. I shall briefly restate my hypothesis: auto-erotism and narcissism include the love for and relation with the internalized good object which in phantasy forms part of the loved body and self. It is to this internalized object that in auto-erotic gratification and narcissistic *states* a withdrawal takes place. Concurrently, from birth onwards, a relation to objects, primarily the mother (her breast) is present. This hypothesis contradicts Freud's concept of auto-erotic and narcissistic *stages* which preclude an object-relation However, the difference between Freud's view and my own is less wide than appears at first sight, since Freud's statements on this issue are not unequivocal. In various contexts he explicitly and implicitly expressed opinions which suggested a relation to an object, the mother's breast, *preceding* auto-erotism and narcissism. One reference must suffice; in the first of two Encyclopaedia articles,[2] Freud said:

> In the first instance the oral component instinct finds satisfaction by attaching itself to the sating of the desire for nourishment; and its object is the mother's breast. It then detaches itself, becomes independent and at the same time *auto-erotic*, that is, it finds an object in the child's own body.

Freud's use of the term object is here somewhat different from my use of this term, for he is referring to the object of an instinctual aim, while I mean, in addition to this, an object-relation involving the infant's emotions, phantasies, anxieties, and defences. Nevertheless, in the sentence referred to, Freud clearly speaks of a libidinal attachment to an object, the mother's breast, which precedes auto-erotism and narcissism.

In this context I wish to remind you also of Freud's findings about early identifications. In *The Ego and the Id,*[3] speaking of abandoned object cathexes, he said; ". . . . the effects of the first identification in earliest childhood will be profound and lasting. This leads us back to the origin of the ego-ideal. . . ." Freud then defines the first and most important identifications which lie hidden behind the ego-ideal as the identification with the father, or with the parents, and places them, as he expresses it, in the "pre-history of every person." These formulations come close to what I described as the first introjected objects, for by definition identifications are the result of introjection. From the statement I have just discussed and the passage quoted from the Encyclopaedia article it can be deduced that Freud, although he did not pursue this line of thought further, did assume that in earliest infancy both an object and introjective processes play a part.

That is to say, as regards auto-erotism and narcissism we meet with an inconsistency in Freud's views. Such inconsistencies which exist on a number of points of theory clearly show, I think, that on these particular issues Freud had not yet arrived at a final decision. In respect of the theory of anxiety he stated this explicitly in *Inhibitions, Symptoms and Anxiety.*[4] His realization that much about the

2. "Psycho-Analysis," 1922. Contained in *Collected Papers*, 5, p. 119.

3. P. 39. On the same page Freud suggests—still referring to these first identifications—that they are a direct and immediate identification which takes place earlier than any object cathexis. This suggestion seems to imply that introjection even precedes object-relations.

4. 1926. Chapter 8, p. 96.

early stages of development was still unknown or obscure to him is also exemplified by his speaking of the first years of the girl's life as ". . . . lost in a past so dim and shadowy . . . ."[5]

I do not know Anna Freud's view about this aspect of Freud's work. But, as regards the question of auto-erotism and narcissism, she seems only to have taken into account Freud's conclusion that an auto-erotic and a narcissistic stage precede object-relations, and not to have allowed for the other possibilities implied in some of Freud's statements such as the ones I referred to above. This is one of the reasons why the divergence between Anna Freud's conception and my conception of early infancy is far greater than that between Freud's views, taken as a whole, and my views. I am stating this because I believe it is essential to clarify the extent and nature of the differences between the two schools of psycho-analytic thought represented by Anna Freud and myself. Such clarification is required in the interests of psycho-analytic training and also because it could help to open up fruitful discussions between psycho-analysts and thereby contribute to a greater general understanding of the fundamental problems of early infancy.

The hypothesis that a stage extending over several months precedes object-relations implies that—except for the libido attached to the infant's own body—impulses, phantasies, anxieties, and defences either are not present in him, or are not related to an object, that is to say they would operate *in vacuo.* The analysis of very young children has taught me that there is no instinctual urge, no anxiety situation, no mental process which does not involve objects, external or internal; in other words, object-relations are at the *center* of emotional life. Furthermore, love and hatred, phantasies, anxieties, and defences are also operative from the beginning and are *ab initio* indivisibly linked with object-relations. This insight showed me many phenomena in a new light.

I shall now draw the conclusion on which the present paper rests: I hold that transference originates in the same processes which in the earliest stages determine object-relations. Therefore we have to go back again and again in analysis to the fluctuations between objects, loved and hated, external and internal, which dominate early infancy. We can fully appreciate the interconnection between positive and negative transferences only if we explore the early interplay between love and hate, and the vicious circle of aggression, anxieties, feelings of guilt and increased aggression, as well as the various aspects of objects towards whom these conflicting emotions and anxieties are directed. On the other hand, through exploring these

5. 1931. "Female Sexuality", contained in *Collected Papers*, 5, p. 254.

early processes I became convinced that the analysis of the negative transference, which had received relatively little attention[6] in psycho-analytic technique, is a precondition for analyzing the deeper layers of the mind. The analysis of the negative as well as of the positive transference and of their interconnection is, as I have held for many years, an indispensable principle for the treatment of all types of patients, children and adults alike. I have substantiated this view in most of my writings from 1927 onwards.

This approach, which in the past made possible the psycho-analysis of very young children, has in recent years proved extremely fruitful for the analysis of schizophrenic patients. Until about 1920 it was assumed that schizophrenic patients were incapable of forming a transference and therefore could not be psycho-analyzed. Since then the psycho-analysis of schizophrenics has been attempted by various techniques. The most radical change of view in this respect, however, has occurred more recently and is closely connected with the greater knowledge of the mechanisms, anxieties, and defences operative in earliest infancy. Since some of these defences, evolved in primal object-relations against both love and hatred, have been discovered, the fact that schizophrenic patients are capable of developing both a positive and a negative transference has been fully understood; this finding is confirmed if we consistently apply in the treatment of schizophrenic patients[7] the principle that it is as necessary to analyze the negative as the positive transference—that in fact the one cannot be analyzed without the other.

Retrospectively it can be seen that these considerable advances in technique are supported in psycho-analytic theory by Freud's discovery of the Life and Death instincts, which has fundamentally added to the understanding of the origin of ambivalence. Because the Life and Death instincts, and therefore love and hatred, are at bottom in the closest interaction, negative and positive transference are basically interlinked.

The understanding of earliest object-relations and the processes they imply has essentially influenced technique and various angles. It has long been known that the psycho-analyst in the transference situation may stand for mother, father, or other people, that he is also at times playing in the patient's mind the part of the superego,

6. This was largely due to the undervaluation of the importance of aggression.

7. This technique is illustrated by H. Segal's paper, "Some Aspects of the Analysis of a Schizophrenic" (*Int. J. Psycho-Anal.*, 31, 1950), and H. Rosenfeld's papers, "Notes on the Psycho-Analysis of the Super-ego Conflict of an Acute Schizophrenic Patient" (*Int. J. Psycho-Anal.*, 33, 1952) and "Transference Phenomena and Transference Analysis in an Acute Catatonic Schizophrenic Patient."

at other times that of the id or the ego. Our present knowledge enables us to penetrate to the specific details of the various roles allotted by the patient to the analyst. There are in fact very few people in the young infant's life, but he feels them to be a multitude of objects because they appear to him in different aspects. Accordingly, the analyst may at a given moment represent a part of the self, of the superego or any one of a wide range of internalized figures. Similarly it does not carry us far enough if we realize that the analyst stands for the actual father or mother, unless we understand which aspect of the parents has been revived. The picture of the parents in the patient's mind has in varying degrees undergone distortion through the infantile processes of projection and idealization, and has often retained much of its phantastic nature. Altogether, in the young infant's mind every external experience is interwoven with his phantasies and on the other hand every phantasy contains elements of actual experience, and it is only by analyzing the transference situation to its depth that we are able to discover the past both in its realistic and phantastic aspects. It is also the origin of these fluctuations in earliest infancy which accounts for their strength in the transference, and for the swift changes—sometimes even within one session—between father and mother, between omnipotently kind objects and dangerous persecutors, between internal and external figures. Sometimes the analyst appears simultaneously to represent both parents—in that case often in a hostile alliance against the patient, whereby the negative transference acquires great intensity. What has then been revived or has become manifest in the transference is the mixture in the patient's phantasy of the parents as one figure, the "combined parent figure" as I described it elsewhere.[8] This is one of the phantasy formations characteristic of the earliest stages of the Oedipus complex and which, if maintained in strength, is detrimental both to object-relations and sexual development. The phantasy of the combined parents draws its force from another element of early emotional life—i.e. from the powerful envy associated with frustrated oral desires. Through the analysis of such early situations we learn that in the baby's mind when he is frustrated (or dissatisfied from inner causes) his frustration is coupled with the feeling that another object (soon represented by the father) receives from the mother the coveted gratification and love denied to himself at that moment. Here is one root of the phantasy that the parents are combined in an everlasting mutual gratification of an oral, anal, and genital nature. And this is in my view the prototype of situations of both envy and jealousy.

8. See *Psycho-Analysis of Children*, particularly Chapters 8 and 11.

There is another aspect of the analysis of transference which needs mentioning. We are accustomed to speak of the transference *situation*. But do we always keep in mind the fundamental importance of this concept? It is my experience that in unravelling the details of the transference it is essential to think in terms of *total situations* transferred from the past into the present, as well as of emotions, defences, and object-relations.

For many years—and this is up to a point still true today—transference was understood in terms of direct references to the analyst in the patient's material. My conception of transference as rooted in the earliest stages of development and in deep layers of the unconscious is much wider and entails a technique by which from the whole material presented the *unconscious elements* of the transference are deduced. For instance, reports of patients about their everyday life, relations, and activities not only give an insight into the functioning of the ego, but also reveal—if we explore their unconscious content—the defences against the anxieties stirred up in the transference situation. For the patient is bound to deal with conflicts and anxieties re-experienced towards the analyst by the same methods he used in the past. That is to say, he turns away from the analyst as he attempted to turn away from his primal objects; he tries to split the relation to him, keeping him either as a good or as a bad figure; he deflects some of the feelings and attitudes experienced towards the analyst on to other people in his current life, and this is part of "acting out."[9]

In keeping with my subject matter, I have predominantly discussed here the earliest experiences, situations, and emotions from which transference springs. On these foundations, however, are built the later object-relations and the emotional and intellectual developments which necessitate the analyst's attention no less than the earliest ones; that is to say, our field of investigation covers *all* that lies between the current situation and the earliest experiences. In fact it is not possible to find access to earliest emotions and object-relations except by examining their vicissitudes in the light of later developments. It is only by linking again and again (and that means hard and patient work) later experiences with earlier ones and *vice versa*, it is only by consistently exploring their interplay, that present and past can come together in the patient's mind. This is one aspect of the process of integration which, as the analysis progresses, en-

9. The patient may at times try to escape from the present into the past rather than realize that his emotions, anxieties, and phantasies are at the time operative in full strength and focused on the analyst. At other times, as we know, the defences are mainly directed against re-experiencing the past in relation to the original objects.

compasses the whole of the patient's mental life. When anxiety and guilt diminish and love and hate can be better synthesized, splitting processes—a fundamental defence against anxiety—as well as repressions lessen while the ego gains in strength and coherence; the cleavage between idealized and persecutory objects diminishes; the phantastic aspects of objects lose in strength; all of which implies that unconscious phantasy life—less sharply divided off from the unconscious part of the mind—can be better utilized in ego activities, with a consequent general enrichment of the personality. I am touching here on the *differences*—as contrasted with the similarities—between transference and the first object-relations. These differences are a measure of the curative effect of the analytic procedure.

I suggested above that one of the factors which bring about the repetition compulsion is the pressure exerted by the earliest anxiety situations. When persecutory and depressive anxiety and guilt diminish, there is less urge to repeat fundamental experiences over and over again, and therefore early patterns and modes of feelings are maintained with less tenacity. These fundamental changes come about through the consistent analysis of the transference; they are bound up with a deep-reaching revision of the earliest object-relations and are reflected in the patient's current life as well as in the altered attitudes towards the analyst.

REFERENCES

1. Freud, Sigmund (1905). 'Fragment of an Analysis of a Case of Hysteria,' *Collected Papers*, 3.
   ——— (1922). 'Psycho-Analysis,' *Collected Papers*, 5.
   ——— (1923). *The Ego and the Id.*
   ——— (1926). *Inhibitions, Symptoms and Anxiety.*
   ——— (1931). 'Female Sexuality,' *Collected Papers*, 5.
2. Klein, Melanie (1932). *The Psycho-Analysis of Children*. Hogarth Press.
   ——— (1946). 'Notes on Some Schizoid Mechanisms,' *Int. J. Psycho-Anal.*, 27, also contained in *Developments in Psycho-Analysis*, by Melanie Klein, Paula Heimann, Susan Isaacs, and Joan Riviere. (London: Hogarth Press, 1952.)
   ——— (1948). *Contributions to Psycho-Analysis, 1921-45.* Hogarth Press.
3. Rosenfeld, Herbert (1952). 'Notes on the Psycho-Analysis of the Super-ego Conflict of an Acute Schizophrenic Patient,' *Int. J. Psycho-Anal.*, 33.
   ——— (1952). 'Transference Phenomena and Transference Analysis in an Acute Catatonic Schizophrenic Patient' (this volume).
4. Segal, Hanna (1950). 'Some Aspects of the Analysis of a Schizophrenic,' *Int. J. Psycho-Anal.*, 31.

2

SASHA NACHT

Silence as an Integrative Factor

Psycho-analytic treatment depends, as we know, on certain exchanges which develop between the patient and his physician, exchanges which are at the same time evoked and limited by what we call the analytic situation.

But is not all exchange between human beings, no matter on what level, based on speech? And is speech not a kind of bridge between two human beings, a bridge by which they can communicate? Furthermore, does not psychoanalytic technique specifically depend on these verbal exchanges? The patient speaks, the doctor comments or interprets, and the insights, center of therapeutic action, result from the interpretations.

This constant exchange between the patient and the physician, these reactions and inter-reactions which form the very woof of psycho-analytic treatment, are possible only through words, spoken words, which bring to the surface the affects which are stirring below: no one has ever thought of carrying on genuine psycho-analytic treatment by mail; the idea itself is absurd.

But why do we think it absurd? Why are we certain that it would not be possible for us to give sufficiently effective explanations and interpretations to someone who outlines in writing his difficulties and conflicts, or relates his dreams even in the greatest detail? The answer will immediately be that the keystone of psycho-analytic treatment is free association of ideas, possible only through speech which almost without conscious effort brings to the surface the buried affects, to which I referred earlier.

Reprinted with permission of the author from the *International Journal of Psychoanalysis,* Vol. 45, 1964, 299-303.

To this reason, sufficient by itself, I will add another: that the psycho-analytic relationship is based on living speech and cannot do without it, unlike other relationships—friendly, intellectual, even perhaps loving relationships—which can sometimes content themselves for many years with contact through the written word.

Here then are the physician and his patient settled in the analytic situation, and allowing a relationship to develop on the basis of a dialogue. Thanks to this relationship, the patient will have an unusual inner experience; we know he will relive in the present a stubbornly-clinging past, of which he is both aware and unaware. He will capture its elusive secrets at work, on the wing; in this sense it is a unique experience.

Each of us, I think, has at one time or another in his career focused his attention on the special nature of the analytic relationship. What is there in this relationship which makes it unique? Everything has been said—and much has been written—on transference, counter—transference, and their manifestations. And yet, in the course of my personal clinical experience, I have often had the impression that an element in this relationship eluded all expression, since often the exchanges between patient and analyst were on a level where speech no longer took place. I came to ask myself these questions: Are there communications which words allow and even foster, and others which it perhaps prevents? Are some affects born from speech, while others can flourish only in silence? I sensed beyond verbal exchanges certain overtones which I could not clearly define and which nevertheless appeared very real to me, as though the analytical relationship was developing on parallel levels, one verbal and the other non-verbal.

In 1957, at the Paris Congress,[1] I already maintained, in the course of the discussion on "Variations in Technique", that therapeutic psycho-analysis did not depend upon interpretations alone, nor therefore on exclusively verbal exchange. The paper which I gave later in Edinburgh[2] in 1961 dealt with the same pre-occupations: discussing "Curative Factors in Psycho-Analysis", I emphasized the effect of the deep inner attitudes of the analyst on the progress of therapy. These seemed to me even more decisive than his interventions and his formulated interpretations. For some time I have been insisting on the primary importance of the role played by the actual unconscious attitude underlying the conscious attitude of the therapist, because of the exchanges which develop beyond words between

1. Nacht, S. (1958). "Variations in Technique." *Int. J. Psycho-Anal.*, 39; *Rev. franc. psychanal.*, 22.

2. Nacht, S. (1962). "Curative Factors in Psycho-Analysis." *Int. J. Psycho-Anal.*, 43; *Rev. franc. psychanal.*, 26.

the unconscious of the physician and that of the patient, and vice versa. This exchange, this communication from unconscious to unconscious, seems to me to find its level at the pre-object phase of the development of the person. This introduces in the relationship an element hard to define, since what the human being feels at this stage cannot be expressed in words; we know that during the first few months of life the object is still not perceived as separate from the self; the subject feels fused in an undifferentiated union with the object.

The nonverbal relationship which appears at moments in the analytic situation seems to me to belong to the state characteristic of that pre-object stage which marks the development of the individual just as much as later phases of ego-development. Some people will always have deep within themselves an unconscious nostalgia for the pre-object stage which is actually the hope of finding it again. That, therefore, is why we will often note the presence of two opposite tendencies: the urge to *separate* oneself from the object, and thus to be *free,* and a concrete urge to achieve complete union with this same object.

The subject finds these drives present just as strongly in the transference relationship during the course of analysis. But the wish for fusion is not verbalized, and is thus harder to detect. It cannot be verbalized, first of all because it is unconscious, of course, and then because its roots are buried in the deepest part of the pre-object level where subject was interchangeable with object. We know that the immaturity of an infant's neurological system until he is 6 months old, so characteristic of the human species, delays his ego development to the time when he can distinguish between subject and object. It seems important to remind ourselves at this point that the first attempts of the ego to function, and the first rudiments of language, make their appearance *at the same time,* i.e. at the very moment when the infant first tries to establish a new method of communication. The ego isolates the subject from the object, and language enhances this separation because it is directed toward this "other." Thus the functions of the ego and those of language agree to sign together the decree of separation which results in the object relationship.

Nevertheless, the language born of this partition will be used by the subject from this point on to try to recapture the object, which is distinct from him, to reach it, to communicate with it; this is the meaning of his first babblings as addressed to the mother. But the subject will never again be able to recapture the state of fusion of the first months of life, a state whose needs linger persistently for many people at their deepest core without touching the conscious.

It is this need which is the basis for the non-verbal relationship in the analytic situation. True transference is first born in the verbal relationship and could not exist without it—but I believe it is the nonverbal relationship which gives it substance and significance during the course of treatment. This nonverbal relationship once born in the silence of the indeterminate, the indefinite, can come to life again only in silence, and that is why certain silences in the course of analysis have seemed to me a necessary condition for the blossoming of an inner state vaguely felt by the patient as *equivalent* to the state of perfect and total union to which he unconsciously aspires. Let us say that he can reach the object from a different angle, yet more *directly* in silence than through speech, because speech is constantly confronted by proofs of the object's remoteness.

What I wish to underline here is the power of this unconscious need for total union in certain human beings. It is not found in the same degree in everyone; some, whose inner interpretation of the experience of separation from the object was felt as liberation, have decisively chosen separation as a way of relating to other people and have found it satisfactory. In contrast, the choice is far less clear-cut for others, who then keep in their lives a vague feeling of incompleteness, a nostalgia which seems to me to be that of a yearning for fusion with the object, which would remove any separation, eliminating all differences. This need for fusion, when it sparks off a search for another approach to awareness, can create great mystics. They, at least, have the privilege of being aware of their urge, and to seek its fulfilment. For the average person, the need remains nebulous, and exists deep within him in a latent state. It deflects inwardly drives which could be used constructively, outwardly in daily life. This is why it seems necessary to me, when this need is too strong because unconscious, that the subject should be enabled to experience it at least fleetingly in analysis, where the nonverbal relationship can allow him to attain (during certain rare moments) a state of inner union with the object-analyst, during which he can enjoy quietness and fulfilment.

I think I can assert from my own clinical experience that if the analyst is vigilant and allows this experience to be so fleeting as to be drained of significance and immediately left behind, and if he resolutely prevents the patient from finding too great satisfaction in it or from seeking purely regressive gratifications, the patient will find, in this brief fulfilment of a profound need, a new peace and strength which will prove invaluable for achieving normal relationships.

Needless to say, in order that this state of union may be beneficial, or even occur, it is necessary for the analyst to have kept the transference as free as possible from aggressive fantasies. This will also keep to a minimum the guilt feelings of the subject. Furthermore—here I make a point which seems to me extremely important and which I have often mentioned—in order that the yearning for fusion can be peacefully experienced by the subject, the object—actually the analyst—must present such an image that total identification with him can be experienced as entirely good and beneficial. He must therefore *be* without qualification, the "good" object who will allow the patient, through an internal process leading to a resolution, to experience an integration of the object so satisfying that he will definitively abandon the regressive phenomenon of transference corresponding to an archaic incorporation, both oral and aggressive, of the analyst. From now on identification with the analyst-object is motivated by a *deep and total acceptance* of him. But, as I have often stressed, to achieve this goal it is essential for the analyst to know how to give up deliberately the rigidity of his customary neutral attitude, so that the subject can feel that the object will be able to welcome, recognize, and accept what the subject finally has become capable of giving. I do not need to emphasize, I believe, that all this must be sensed and perceived by the patient without concrete proof from the analyst of his vigilant interest. The analyst must limit himself to a certain way of being *present* with an underlying, deeply-felt attitude compounded of acceptance, availability, and the sincere desire to help the patient. Only this deep positive attitude can completely reassure the subject; he may detect it in the words of the analyst, but it is certainly even more in the unspoken intangible quality of his presence revealing the real character of the counter-transference that the patient will be able to find the security which he needs so much. If he does not find it, the transference neurosis runs the risk of being melted into a permanently sado-masochistic relationship, and therefore becoming incurable.

On the other hand, because the unconscious wish for union-communion leaves behind the analyst himself, and with him the maternal object, in the search for some unknown primary source of life, the nonverbal relationship with the analyst is in a sense depersonalized and drained of passionate emotion. The object is no longer *utilized* unconsciously, and because of this, the bonds which imprison the patient in the transference neurosis have a tendency to loosen. The almost impersonal character of this primary urge towards union can thus, by the kind of fulfilment lived through during the course of the analysis, help to dispel transference neurosis. This is an important point, if we consider that until this transformation has taken place, no cure can be possible; the neurosis of the patient has simply changed its *aspect*.

I will perhaps be asked: But how does this unconscious drive towards a kind of fusion manifest itself during the course of treatment, and more particularly, what form does the fulfilment take? Here I can only offer the results of my own clinical observation; this need expresses itself by a certain quality of silence which fosters non-verbal relationship between the patient and his physician. In the same way it can occur when the subject, having eliminated fear and aggression, can tolerate a certain enduring silence of authentic peace in the deepest regions of himself, where he *feels* finally not only in agreement but even in communion with the object. In this state, experienced as a kind of oneness, all opposition and all ambivalence lose their sense and their *raison d'êtr.* It is precisely this which allows the patient to accept willingly the integration of the analyst as object, and at the same time all that the analyst has given and taught him. These moments, even though fleeting, are in my opinion very fruitful. They free the patient from an unconscious need which is a source of resistance until it has found a form in which it can be realized.

From now on, the explanations and the interpretations of the analyst will be accepted and experienced altogether differently. The patient is no longer afraid of his own silence, since it is no longer the expression of his discomfort or his resistance. The analyst's verbal interventions will therefore be *received* in a different manner, and if the patient listens to them from his peaceful inner silence, the words will *form roots* in his deepest being and will bear fruit, whereas before they were virtually lost almost as soon as they were heard, swirled along in currents of agitated thought, constantly in turmoil. It is in this sense that silence can play a significant role in the process of integration. Words sow seeds; just as seeds germinate and sprout first in the peaceful silence of the earth, so now in silence and in peace the self grows and develops. And does not psychoanalytic treatment attempt, in the last analysis, to lead a person towards a rebirth in what becomes for him a new world?

In the course of treatment, when attempting to give certain interpretations to the patient, or to evoke in him certain reactions, I have often had the impression that speech was a clumsy tool to use on the fragile mechanisms of the human psyche. Is the language of the unconscious translatable into conscious language, and is not the "translation," more than in other areas, close to a betrayal? In the same way, can the analyst's words, his conscious language, adequately be understood by the patient's unconscious? I think that the analyst often makes the mistake of believing that the words he uses have the *same* value for the patient as for himself. However, language often deforms and distorts certain shifting, subtle meanings which when isolated, defined, given a shape, can become terrifying or grotesque. To put into words certain almost elusive ripples of the unconscious psyche is to give these form and power which can be disturbing to a patient, haunt him and torment him. We all know how certain fantasies, such as those described by Klein, undoubtedly correspond to the content of certain deep levels of the unconscious. But when the analyst interprets to the patient fantasies of a parcelled object which has been swallowed, internalized, absorbed, assimilated, and when he does this again and again, emphasizing them beyond what is strictly indicated, does he not impose on the patient certain images terrifying because their very verbalization makes them so? In addition, we can wonder whether interpretation of fantasies is not sometimes made at the very moment when they begin to lose their effective power. I mean by this that the subject is almost ready to abandon them, and, therefore, the interventions which revive them can only thwart his yearning to be rid of them. Words often give shape to affects which are by themselves extremely fluid, and force them to harden into forms which do not correspond with their essential truth. This is why the analyst must be more vigilant than anyone and must employ words prudently. For example, a few words will suffice when dealing with certain fantasies whose expression is tolerated with difficulty by the patient's conscious. It is better to say little, and to allow a certain silence to occur immediately afterwards during which earlier words will evoke in the unconscious certain *resonances* rather than precise images for the conscious. We could almost say that, in analysis, language has no better assistant than silence, because in silence its full significance and deep efficaciousness is best realized. Similarly, we could also say that the verbal relationship between analyst and patient functions at its optimum only if a certain nonverbal relationship is present concurrently to supplement it by providing overtones and undertones. The ability to reach and to maintain a certain quality of silence influences the quality of the nonverbal relationship in the analytic situation.

Is it really necessary to add that in order that the patient may be able to tolerate silence, the analyst must first be capable of it himself? If certain silences make him even slightly ill at ease, if he feels the need to cough, or to light a cigarette, or to shift his position, the patient will be perfectly aware of his underlying discomfort, and will not be able to let himself go into the deep quietude which he needs so much. Because he is disturbed, the psychoanalyst will then represent a threat to the patient's unconscious. When the analyst is feared, silence becomes resistance. The communication from unconscious to unconscious of which I was speaking has the effect of making the doctor's anxiety not only perceptible to the patient, but also contagious. It therefore seems indispensable to me that the psychoanalyst should be free of unconscious fear, that he should have been able to eliminate fear from his own psyche as much as possible. Anyone who feels fear cannot bear silence anyway. This is why, if certain silences are effective in expressing resistance to treatment, according to classical theory, inability to endure silence seems to me to reveal other forms of resistance located, perhaps, on a more significant level. All silences of patients do not express the same thing, as I have tried to show. Silence, like speech, can mask positive affects or negative ones. It is up to the analyst to comprehend their correct significance, and he will achieve this only if he has been able to allow the patient at moments to establish with him this sort of nonverbal communication, based on perfect peacefulness.

If I specify here that the analyst must permit the patient to establish *at moments* this kind of relationship, it is because it seems to me necessary to insist on the fact that this relationship which allows the patient to attain an inner state of fusion can occur only in certain crucial moments of therapy; the patient must not settle into this state any more than into transference neurosis. Both seem to me indispensable for good progress in treatment provided that the patient is not allowed to cling to them and to find in them delights which he would then become incapable of relinquishing.

It is no doubt beneficial to allow the subject to become aware of the existence of needs on a level *other* than the instinctual drives, but the physician must still emphasize the primary necessity of a wholesome adjustment to the bipolarity of object relationship. This is why, if his own deep-rooted attitudes have allowed the subject to attain at moments an internal form of fusion, for which he was obscurely yearning, the analyst must nevertheless return him immediately on the road to external reality. Thus, the unconscious need for union fleetingly realized during analysis will guide the subject towards the acceptance of the inevitable separation which constitutes good object relation, separation until then felt unconsciously as painful, if not intolerable.

If this is the role of silence in the success of treatment, it is obviously not negligible. For my part, I have been able to attribute to silence a power of integration indispensable to the effectiveness of speech. Actually, does not everything which lives take rise in silence and end in silence too? More specifically, human life needs at moments to steep itself in silence, from which it draws essential nourishment and in which it develops its deepest.

3

M. MASUD R. KHAN

Silence as Communication

Adolescence is not an
affliction but a
normative crisis.
–Erik Erikson (7)

Silence in the analytic situation is a recurrent and complex clinical phenomenon. Recently Arlow (1) and Zeligs (24) have discussed exhaustively the patient's silence as serving the functions of discharge, defense and communication in the analytic situation. Balint (2) has related silence in the clinical analytic situation to primary psychic creativity and creation as they emerge in early ego development.

In my clinical report on the first sixteen sessions from the introductory phase of a male adolescent patient's psychoanalytic treatment, I shall try to show the communicative function of his persistent silence in the analytic situation. In my discussion, I shall not enlarge upon the defensive function of silence either as a defiance of the therapeutic process, or as a typical adolescent flight from intrapsychic conflict. (7, 23) I shall only briefly discuss the discharge function of his silence as seeking a magical symbiotic fusion with the analyst. (10) These elements were present and were interpreted. But it is my contention that from the stage reported in the treatment of this one adolescent patient, it was the judicious withholding of therapeutic intervention, either through excessive interpretation or reassurance, that enabled him to communicate his real inner conflicts and predicament.

I shall try to show the primary function of his silence was to communicate through the transference and the analytic process a very disturbed early childhood relationship to his mother which had brought about identity diffusion (6) at adolescence. The regressive and defiant flight into a negative identity (7) was his private and magical attempt to deal with this developmental predicament. My major

Reprinted from the *Bulletin of the Menninger Clinic*, Vol. 27, 1963, 300-310.

concern is to detail the reconstruction of the cumulative trauma (16) through the analytic process in the treatment of the patient. The cumulative trauma was the sustained, pathogenic encroachment on his childhood developmental processes by the disturbed relationship to his mother. I shall try to show that counter-transference was an instrument for perceiving and deciphering the affectivity and archaic object-relationships as they were expressed by the patient through his silent behaviour in the analytic situation. (12, 22) The persistent silence was also a mode of acting out and served the functions of recollecting, integrating and working through the pathogenic early relationship to the mother. (5, 11, 13)

Almost all analysts have stressed the technical difficulties involved in treating adolescent patients. (3, 4, 8, 9, 17) In the clinical handling of this case I have been guided and helped by the researches of Erikson (6, 7) and Winnicott. (20, 21, 23) When faced with the young patient's adamant refusal to speak, I was profoundly encouraged by a counsel of Winnicott's: "Many treatments of schizoid types of adolescents fail because they are planned on a basis that ignores the child's ability to think up—in a way, to *create*—an analyst, a role into which the real analyst can try to fit himself." (20) Once I had diagnosed that the negativity and withdrawal into inertia and apathy were both an appeal for help and an expression of an antisocial tendency, I was ready to involve the clinical process in an enactment of these intrapsychic conflicts. The chief idiom the patient used to communicate and express these was silence, and it is the clinical handling of this silence that I shall recount.

Case Report

The patient, whom I shall call Peter, was just over eighteen years of age. He had been referred to me by a psychiatrist because of the parents' acute anxiety and concern about the patient. Peter had been progressively withdrawing from his school activities and social interests over the past five years. The climax had been reached when he willfully refused to finish his last paper in a competitive entrance examination and had sat idly doodling and scribbling instead. He had also isolated himself in his room, spending all his time listening to classical music and reading highbrow novels. He rarely went out or spoke to anyone. At home he was polite, but totally aloof and uncommunicative. The presence of psychiatric illness in the family had made the parents anxious for help. They were afraid Peter might deteriorate into an illness of a schizoid-depressive type, or that he might attempt suicide.

By all accounts, Peter was intelligent, alert and gifted, with leanings towards art and literature. Though he had always been shy and sensitive, his behavior had been normal during latency. Until a few years previously, he had enjoyed his school and social life. It had been impressed upon me by the referring psychiatrist that Peter was in urgent need of help, but it would be difficult to get him to accept treatment. One further problem needed immediate attention. He was due to take his high school graduation examination in three months, and the parents dreaded that if he shirked it, and he was likely to because of his avowed refusal to go to a university, then his whole life would be prejudiced and affected by it. The only other facts I knew about Peter before I saw him in consultation were that he came from a professional upper class and had enjoyed good home life. There was little overt conflict with the parents.

The youth who arrived for consultation was an elegant, fragile, polite and polished person. He talked fitfully but thoughtfully and used language with distinctive clarity and correctness. He was neither secretive nor defensively or anxiously hostile. He made it clear that he had come to discuss matters so as not to cause his parents further distress. He had no intention of undertaking analytic treatment because it would be a stupid waste of time. He had been to a psychotherapist the year before and had not been able to talk, so the treatment had to be given up. He did not feel that he was either ill or needed help. He had simply decided not to go on with education and instead to do some ordinary job which would pay enough for him to live and to go to musical concerts. He then asked what I wanted him to do and I suggested he should give the treatment a try. He protested he could come only once a week as he was still attending school an hour a day. We agreed that he should come every Saturday.

What had impressed me most during the consultations were: 1) His capacity for genial and intelligent conversation alongside his negativity and refusal to seek help. I felt he was not so hostile against me and the treatment as engrossed in a very personal mood. 2) His polite and fragile style and a certain static quality about his way of sitting. He had neither moved nor fidgeted even once during the consultation. 3) I could easily distinguish between his polite, social behavior and his private mood of inertia and self-engrossment. 4) Though he could talk lucidly, he had utterly failed to say anything significant about the private withdrawn world he lived in. 5) He had made light of his refusal to do the examination paper. I regarded this as an isolated and impulsive antisocial act through which he had been able to signal and appeal to his parents that he needed help.

I am using the concept of antisocial tendency as defined by Winnicott. (21)

> "The antisocial tendency is characterized by *an element in it which compels the environment to be important.* The patient through unconscious drives compels someone to attend to management . . . *The antisocial tendency implies hope* . . . when there is an antisocial tendency *there has been a true deprivation* . . . that is to say, there has been a loss of something good that has been positive in the child's experience up to a certain date, and that has been withdrawn; the withdrawal has extended over a period of time longer than that over which the child can keep the memory of the experience alive (Cf. Shields [18]).

I decided that since the patient had been able to communicate his predicament only through an antisocial act, it was very important to concentrate on enabling him to express his withdrawn mood in the analytic situation and through the analytic process. I decided to use the classical analytic procedure (recumbent position and verbal free associations) and totally refrain from any guidance of or involvement with his family, his school difficulties and approaching examination. I felt that his withdrawn mood of inertia, his refusal to finish his examination paper, and his belief that he would not be able to speak in the analytic situation, were expressions of some basic need and conflict in him. From the very beginning he found it hard to speak. He was obviously anxious and afraid that I would adopt an incriminating attitude. From what little he said during the first four sessions, I gathered that his personal life had come to a standstill and he lived in a hopeless state of inertia and apathy, consoled by his music and excessive reading of novels.

The experience and observation of this silent state was more arduous than I had anticipated. I persisted, however, in letting the clinical process take its own course and shape and evolve its pattern according to the patient's needs. This entailed literally living through his silences with him and experiencing every nuance of his body-behavior and mood-atmosphere. Even though the completely silent sessions were six in number, it is important to bear in mind that the time involved was six weeks. It was important for him that I could bear the strain and anxiety from it and did not directly contact his parents. After the first four sessions, Peter became utterly mute, silent and frozen. I am distinguishing muteness from silence here. Muteness, I felt, had a destructive, aggressive, belligerent tone to it, whereas silence was a more benign or neutral state. I shall now discuss some of the salient features of his mute, silent and frozen behavior and its relation to his childhood traumatic experiences.

Soon it became clear that the silent state was a complex one. The great difficulty was about knowing precisely what was happening and when. I could sense and feel in his body-tensions, in his posture, and facial expressions, a continuous flux of feelings and attitudes.

The first inference important for me was that the patient was enacting a state of affectivity, in which two people are involved and yet each was a "creation" of the other. Describing the area of "basic fault" Balint (2) states, "The force originating from the basic fault has not the form of a conflict." I felt strongly that the patient was not in conflict with me. It felt more like a state in which two people who could be alive and responsive to each other had become frozen and petrified by each other. The patient expected me magically to free him from his frozen state, just as I expected him to speak so that I could help him. There was an archaic affectivity involved which Peter's adult ego functions could not express or communicate. In the analytic situation silence and nonverbalization were the vehicle of this mood and affectivity. These emotions and affects, though they were loosely enveloped in his mood and attitude of frozen passivity, inertia, and silence, could, however, be registered sentiently by me as varying from pleasant well-being and liveliness to sullen anger, muted rage and helpless despondency.

Gradually I began to realize, through the impact of the silences on me and my inner reactions to them, that Peter was using me as his auxiliary ego. He was making me experience and register what he had lived through passively at some stage of his development. I was the child Peter, and he was the other person from the original childhood situation. I could sense in my role as child-Peter that he must have felt reduced to impotence, futility and exhaustion through the mood and behavior of this other person, just as I was experiencing these now through him. I learned that to be seduced into hopeful liveliness and expectancy because he looked alert and perky on arrival was a sure way of experiencing painful rejection during the rest of the session. The more I felt responsive and expected responsiveness from Peter, the more bitterly futile and helpless I felt at the end of the session.

One striking feature of these silences was that they were not directed against me in any hostile and viciously vindictive way. It was essentially a question of his being engrossed in a deadly depressive inert state and my having to share it. Of course there were oscillations of mood. He only became hostile or bloody-minded when I would verbally intrude on his silence with persistent interpretations.

The next thing I realized was that through these *silences* Peter was presenting me with "another person." This other person he had experienced and registered with singular vividness across a long period of time. I began to infer that this person must have suffered from acute depression and had consequently felt apathetic and inert in relation to the child-Peter.

Watching my personal reaction to his silence, I was impressed by how often I was impelled to *nudge* him physically. Of course I never did. But the wish was there; and the illusion that this would make him come alive and react responsively and feelingly was very strong in me. When trapped in the long, intense and bleak deadness of some of his silences, I always had the wish in me somehow to rattle him into liveliness. The greatest temptation I had to fight against in myself, during these moments, was to *act on him* through verbal interpretations.

I had found out from experience that if I started to give some interpretation *e.g.* that he was testing me, provoking me or attacking me with his silences, then his mood would change. He would become sullen, his body-tone would flop and all one had was a collapsed heap of a boy on the couch.

Another important element in the relationship that was being reenacted in the transference was the positive bond with and attachment to the person. I had been impressed with the punctuality and regularity with which Peter attended his sessions. He had to travel a long way, and it was a strain on him. This I inferred repeated a positive libidinal bond to the person in the original childhood situation. There was never any doubt about his wish to come to the sessions. This also made me pursue the latent meaning and logic of his silences more seriously rather than interpret them exclusively as resistance only.

There was a distinct affect of pain, loss and dejection to the silences. It was difficult to differentiate the phenomenology of his silent moods. Feelings and processes changed so rapidly, invisibly and yet sentiently. At one moment I was child-Peter feeling his reactions; and the next he would be child-Peter in his own right lying helpless and sullen. The most important thing clinically was to distinguish the role of the analytic transference process between Peter and me from the existence and role of Peter and me as persons in the analytic setting. The analytic setting enabled this regressive reenactment of the childhood experience. This peculiar and specific mode of "remembering" involved child-Peter and me, but was sustained and made possible by the analytic setting. To try and introduce notions of interpersonal conflict between Peter and me was always disruptive at this stage. It was also clear that in this reenacted affectivity and mood, Peter in the role of this other person imposed a task upon me which I had no option but to bear with. He had no capacity to meet my expectancy, namely to talk and free associate which I inferred must have been true of the original situation. He had put up with the other person's depression while that person had not been able to meet the patient's needs and aliveness. (11, 19, 22)

Observing my reactions to his silent mood, I concluded that

Peter's traumata in childhood must have been in terms of his lively expectations and wishes to engage this person in excited, aggressive interchange. The evidence for this was that if I felt tired at some point in the session or disinclined to concentrate on his mood and wandered off in my thinking, I felt no strain. There was only his idle, dull presence on the couch. It was only my alive responsiveness and expectancy that made his silence into a torture of frustration, futility, anger, and despondency for me.

My role and function during his silences was to provide a sentient, concentrated alert attention. This attention had to be more than merely listening. It is listening with one's mind and body. If my attention sagged, or I got the slightest bit bored and tired, the clinical process immediately lost its vitality. The important element in this body attention was the capacity to utilize neutralized, aggressive cathexes in one's attention on the patient. (14)

It is important to stress here that during the six silent sessions only the patient had been silent. I had sparingly, but regularly, commented on whatever I could put together by way of inference about his shifts of mood and feelings in the sessions, from observing his behavior. I always made some summary, brief comment at the end of each silent session. To Peter this indicated that I had been watching and participant in the situation. It also established my separateness from him and provided a verbal link with the next session. The linking function of these interpretations was important, as we were to discover fully in retrospect later in his treatment. To Peter it had meant that another person, who was not he, could empathize with his state of mind and feelings, without his either being overwhelmed by them or subsumed by them. My behavior provided a model for reality testing in the analytic situation, both in establishing separateness between him and me as two persons in the situation and in discriminating between fantasy (inner reality) and external reality.

Through these brief statements about his feelings, it became possible for Peter to learn that what another person says and does can change one's mood, that people can help and communicate with each other, and magical incorporations or archaic fusions with objects are not the only way of dealing with emotional relationships. I was, of course, only relatively correct and accurate in my statements about his moods and feelings. It was important to indicate that feelings can be perceived and talked about instead of being *lived* and acted out. Another aspect of my providing Peter with verbalization was that it proved that I was not retaliating against his silence with silence, that I could tolerate the hostile and rejective elements in his silence without being threatened by them. Through my verbalization (interpretation) of his feelings, I lent him my ego-function to test his inner reality. Thus, he could gradually relax his magical and archaic defenses.

One of the easiest errors to make when either irritated or exhausted by the strain and stress of Peter's silence was to give interpretations that would provoke guilt or sound reproachful. It was, however, important to keep myself aware of the reproachfulness that his behavior provoked in me. It is my contention that every nuance of feeling that I experienced in relation to his silences was in some form or another his own experience in the original traumatic relationship.

Present in Peter's persistent attitude of silence and withdrawal was also a diffuse state of excitement in him. I could sense it in his body-tone and posture on the couch. I felt that he had invented a new idiom of being where he had projected all his own excitement to "external" things, like music and fictional characters. He lived passively surrounded by these. Even intrapsychically he lived at a distance from his thoughts and preoccupations. This recreation of a pure pleasure-self fed by music and literature had a protective function as well as a discharge function. It protected him and the other person (in analysis, me) from his reactive sadism and aggression. How his mother's depression must have exaggerated the sadistic rage reactions in the frustrated child I could infer from the amount of aggressive feelings his silence and inertia roused in me. It was also clear that the withdrawn state defended the self and the object against aggression. One consequence of this was that of paralyzing the ego-functions and a reactive idealization of primitive pleasure.

From these, and myriad other fleeting impressions, observations and inferences, I decided to interpret to Peter what I thought were the content and meaning of his withdrawal state and silence in analysis. This I did in the eleventh session (roughly three months after the start of the treatment and after the sixth silent session). I interpreted to him that observing his behavior, and the mood-relationship he had involved me in through his silences, I was left in little doubt that he had experienced in his childhood relation to his mother over a considerable length of time, what he was repeating in the analytic situation; that his mother had suffered from a severe depression in which he had been helplessly involved. This had imposed a strain on him, especially in relation to his lively, aggressive, contact-seeking impulses. He had reacted by becoming passive, despondent and depressed. In time it had all changed and he had been absorbed in the routine processes of growth, development and socialization.

At puberty and adolescence when he had to define his own aims and ideals and find his new role as a sexual adult male, the whole conflict had reemerged and he had to get back to the original relationship to sort it out. He had tried to invent a totally new identity for himself through absorption with music and identification with various fictional characters. In fact, he had tried to discover a new milieu where he *became* what he read. This was an as-if identity, which aimed at recreating an idealized pleasure-ego, unrelated to reality and free of all conflict. He denuded himself of all emotions and contacts and lived surrounded by music. This enabled him to deny, both his *actual* need to be dependent on his parents, and the need to be nursed through the original trauma and its sequelae. The addiction to music served as a denial of his despair, dependency-needs and wish to cry and scream. He had been also scared that his magical attempt at a new concocted identity might succeed all too well.

His parents, because of their knowledge of the mother's depression in his childhood, had felt guilty and responsible and, therefore, had been all too permissive and accommodating toward his withdrawal techniques. Hence he had to act out through refusing to finish his entrance examination paper to compel them to seek therapeutic intervention on his behalf. What he was seeking was a setting and relationship in which both dependency-needs and aggression could be integrated. The refusal was both an appeal and an act directed against the destructive regressive strength of his withdrawal techniques. This act had exposed him to full view and his family could see he was ill. Similarly, silence in the sessions was a way of *showing*. In regressive mood, magical gestures were his only idiom of communication.

I was rather surprised when Peter reacted to this long construction with the remarks that he remembered his mother's depression all too well. He was then about three years of age. He could time and place it, because Jenny, the young girl who had been looking after him and the other children, had begun to play a progressively more important role in his life and that of the family. She had, more or less, taken over the management of the household. She was still with them, and she was the only person he had been able to talk to with any spontaneity for the past five years. He had a notion that his mother had gone in for a lengthy analytic treatment.

Then he was silent for a long while. He broke his silence by volunteering to tell me a dream. It was not a new dream. He had dreamed it first when he was six years old and it has recurred in different variations since, though not during the past five years. The dream was: "I am in my grandmother's house by the seaside. A crab is trying to come through the glass window. I feel very threatened and frightened and wake up screaming." I interpreted that the crab signified his own aggressive aliveness and excitement which he had repressed and could experience only as a threat. In association to the dream he added that his mother had the next child after him around that time. He thought perhaps he had been sent away when she was due to have the baby.

It was clear from this that when the mother had recovered from her depression, she had another child and gradually family life had returned to normal. But in between, Peter had dissociated his aliveness and agressive vitality. This had enabled him to be a delicate, sensitive and compliant boy during latency. It was only with the resurgence of instinctuality at puberty and the need to integrate his inner resources, that he had found himself facing the original traumata. Then he had tried the solution by withdrawal and the invention of a private, regressive pleasure–self screened by his negative social identity. I communicated most of this to Peter. When Peter came for the next session he looked more lively and eager to talk. He asked me whether his father had been in touch with me. He told me that he had let them know he was going in for the examination in two week's time. I was deeply relieved to hear this. He must have sensed this because he remarked: "Don't get too hopeful. I have not promised to go to the university."

Peter wanted to take the next week off for the preparation for the examination and I let him. He took the examination. I saw him once again before the summer break. He wanted to think over the whole question of the treatment and decide for himself about it. I agreed to this too.

I saw Peter after six weeks. He had been miserable and unhappy. This he said was a change from being dead and inert. He had passed the examination all right. He told me that his father had asked him to discuss what he was going to do about going to the university. He asked me what was he to do? I replied it all depended on how he felt. He said he could now see that the idea of refusing education was merely a way of getting back at the parents and, therefore, he was no longer against going to the university on principle. He could not, however, face going there and doing all the work and being caught up in all the activities. He had felt depressed during the holidays and "damned near to a breakdown." He also said: "My parents' fear that I might commit suicide is not that much of a myth. Only I do not even know what I will be killing myself for." He also said he was willing to go in for full treatment.

I told Peter that I agreed with him that going to the university would be a useless and disruptive strain on him. What he needed was a setting to be ill in. I said I would talk to his father and see whether the issue of the university could be postponed for a year. Then he would be in a better position to decide. Meantime he could live at home if he wished. He agreed to all this.

Peter's father, when I saw him, was quite cooperative about all my suggestions. He said he had known all along Peter would have a breakdown since he had been all too compliant and goody-goody throughout childhood, while the elder brother had shown severe symptoms. The father was also instinctively aware of the effect of the mother's depression on Peter. He added one significant fact, however. Five years previously the father had been taken seriously ill with a heart complaint. We agreed that Peter should stay at home. I warned the father that Peter could become seriously depressed and ill in which case he would have to be hospitalized. The father understood this also and was willing to cooperate.

I shall only briefly recount that Peter sank into a deep regressive state for some five months. During this period he stayed either in bed most of the day listening to music and reading, or just sitting idle and staring. He came five times a week regularly for treatment. During the regressive period he could not bear any relation with his mother and everything was done for him by Jenny, his childhood nurse. The parents were most patient and understanding and neither intruded upon him nor spoiled him.

In analysis we were now able to work verbally through reactions of loss, grief and rage in reaction to the mother's depression. Gradually he started to reemerge and wish to do things. He tried a few things, but could not sustain his interest or effort. He tried skating and kept at it. I have not the space available to discuss the strange way this youth found his way back to mobility and aliveness through skating. In another four months he felt inclined to study again and went to the university after the summer, where he did well the first year he was there. A recent dream of his showed clearly how much his internal emotional situation has changed. He dreamed about a pretty classmate of his: "We are sitting in the canteen. She comes over, leans her head against my shoulder and starts to cry. I was able to comfort her and she began to smile."

Peter had felt very pleased he had been able to dream this dream. (15) To him it meant that he had begun to believe that he could change another person's mood and feelings. In the dream it was the girl's feelings, intrapsychically it meant the mother's as well. He now felt that there could be mutual responsiveness and communication with another person, and he did not have to magically internalize all emotional states in order to deal with them. He stressed his relief that he could recognize depression outside himself in another person. He felt this gave him freedom and the ability to do something about it. From here the theme of the value of mourning and sharing sadness emerged. He felt related to others.

The dream was also an attempt to replace the incestuous object (mother) by a new, contemporary one. This he felt freed him to be friends with his mother once again. He had always admired his mother and now would not have to persist with negating her presence at home and denying his genuinely affectionate feelings for her. Altogether Peter had felt very positive on waking up. The dream, he said, had given him a new freedom and a new start.

Conclusion

Erikson (7) in discussing the therapeutic problems encountered in the clinical handling of identity-diffusion in adolescents, details "a phase of particular malignancy" and "the rock-bottom attitude" which accompanies the search for "the ultimate limit of regression and the only firm foundation for a renewed progression." He relates these to Kris's concept of "regression in the service of the ego." Winnicott (23) discusses pertinently "the close relationship that exists between the normal difficulties of adolescence and the abnormality that may be called the antisocial tendency." In my clinical report I have discussed:

1. An adolescent's retreat into negative identity and identity diffusion. (7)
2. In this context, the function of antisocial tendency (21) as an appeal for help as well as an expression of the early failure of the mother in relation to the child's ego-needs.
3. The acting out of the antisocial tendency in transference and analytic setting through persistent silence.
4. The function of this silence to communicate the patient's disturbed relation to the mother in childhood.
5. The use of countertransference perceptions of the analytic process and the patient's transference to decipher the nature, and meaning of this disturbed mother-child relationship in the patient.
6. The reconstruction of the cumulative trauma in this patient's childhood as it was repeated in his silence through the transference and analytic process and its interpretations to the patient.
7. By allowing the patient's silence full expressive scope in the analytic situation, I enabled him to "create" out of me and the analytic process a clinical idiom through which he could reenact and communicate the affectivity and unconscious conflicts relating to his mother's depression in his childhood and his involvement with these.
8. The reconstruction of the cummulative trauma in relation to the mother's depression in childhood and its working through led to the gradual release of his capacities to use positively regression to dependence in the service of the ego, and enabled him to re-discover his spontaneity, initiative and the capacity to live and work in his contemporary milieu creatively.

REFERENCES

1. Arlow, J. A.: "Silence and the Theory of Technique." *J. Amer. Psa. Assn.* 9:44-55, 1961.
2. Balint, Michael: The Three Areas of the Mind. *Int. J. Psa.* 39:328-340, 1958.
3. Blos, Peter: The Concept of Acting Out in Relation to the Adolescent Process. *J. Amer. Acad. Child Psychiat.* 2:118-143, 1963.
4. Eissler, K. R.: Notes on Problems of Technique in the Psychoanalytic Treatment of Adolescents. *Psa. Study of the Child* 13:223-254, 1958.
5. Ekstein, Rudolf and Friedman, S. W.: Acting Out, Play Action and Play Acting. *J. Amer. Psa. Assn.* 5:581-629, 1957.
6. Erikson, E. H.: *Childhood and Society.* New York, Norton, 1950.
7. _______: The Problem of Ego Identity. *J. Amer. Psa. Assn.* 4:56-121, 1956.
8. Freud, Anna: Adolescence. *Psa. Study of the Child* 12:255-278, 1958.
9. Geleerd, E. R.: Some Aspects of Psychoanalytic Technique in Childhood. *Psa. Study of the Child* 12:263-283, 1957.
10. _______: Some Aspects of Ego Vicissitudes in Adolescence. *J. Amer. Psa. Assn.* 9:394-405, 1961.
11. Greenacre, Phyllis: Problems of Acting Out in the Transference Relationship. *J. Amer. Acad. Child Psychiat.* 2:144-175, 1963.
12. Heimann, Paula: On Counter-Transference. *Int. J. Psa.* 31:81-84, 1950.
13. Kanzer, Mark: Acting Out, Sublimation and Reality Testing. *J. Amer. Psa. Assn.* 5:663-684, 1957.
14. Khan, M. M. R.: Regression and Integration in the Analytic Setting. *Int. J. Psa.* 41:130-146, 1960.
15. _______: Dream Psychology and the Evolution of the Psycho-Analytic Situation. *Int. J. Psa.* 43:21-31, 1962.
16. _______: The Concept of Cumulative Trauma. *Psa. Study of the Child,* Vol. 18, 1963.
17. Spiegel, L. A.: Identity and Adolescence. In *Adolescents*, Sandor Lorand and H. I. Schneer, eds. New York, Hoeber, 1961.
18. Shields, R. W.: *A Cure of Delinquents.* London, Heinemann, 1962.
19. Spitz, R. A.: Transference. *Int. J. Psa.* 37:380-385, 1956.
20. Winnicott, D. W.: Paediatrics and Psychiatry. In *Collected Papers.* New York, Basic Books, 1958, pp. 157-173.
21. _______: The Antisocial Tendency. In *Collected Papers.* New York, Basic Books, 1958, pp. 306-315.
22. _______: Clinical Varieties of Transference. In *Collected Papers.* New York, Basic Books, 1958, pp. 295-299.
23. _______: Adolescence. *The New Era* Vol. 43, No. 8, 1962.
24. Zeligs, M. A.: The Psychology of Silence: Its Role in Transference, Countertransference and the Psychoanalytic Process. *J. Amer. Psa. Assn.* 9:7-43, 1961.

4

ANTONIO J. FERREIRA

On Silence

Who then . . . tells a finer tale than any of us? Silence does. And where does one read a deeper tale than upon the most perfectly printed page of the most precious book? Upon the blank page.

—Isak Dinesen, *Last Tales*

Since the earliest insights into the dynamic aspects of mental life, the silent patient has stimulated a great deal of interest and raised questions of importance to both the theory and practice of psychotherapy. Historically speaking, the problem of silence in psychotherapy has been understood in ways that differed and changed along with the evolving conceptions of the psychotherapeutic process itself.

It has been part of the psychotherapist's heritage to expect the patient to talk, and to regard silence, particularly if repeated or protracted, as an unwelcome development in the course of psychotherapy. As is well known, an early conception of psychotherapy, directly inspired by Charcot's work on hypnosis, placed emphasis on verbalization. With the introduction of the notion of catharsis, the patient was expected to speak out his thoughts, and silence, regarded as resistance and an obstacle to the progress of therapy, was to be discouraged by more or less authoritarian means.

A second conception of psychotherapy grew out of a richer understanding of the mental apparatus and a further realization of the role that symbolism and unconscious processes play in human intercourse. In this light, silence began to be apprehended not just as a resistance to or a gap in the therapeutic flow, but as a symbolic

Reprinted with permission of the author and publisher from the *American Journal of Psychotherapy*, Vol. XVIII, 109-115.

unit in itself as important as the verbal units that preceded or followed it. Although men of letters and popular wisdom had for centuries observed upon the significances of silence—silence as wisdom (1), caution (2), anger (3), joy (4), love (5), scorn (6), and so on—it was not until the advent of psychoanalysis that we began to realize its implications and uncover its meanings in terms of the unconscious. Thus silence came to be recognized as a symbol of death (7), homosexuality (8), aggression (9), oral masturbation (10), anal-erotic pleasure (11), repression of pregenitality (12), displaced punishment (13), and other symbols (14-19).

But slowly, a third conception of psychotherapy was in the making, strongly imbued with the notions of Gestalt, field, and relationship. Within this distinctly different psychotherapeutic framework, the "meaning" of silence became an obsolete question. Silence, like any other happening in psychotherapy, became but an aspect of the multidimensional continuum that characterizes both behavior and emotional life. And although we may continue to investigate its occurrence as a particularly interesting phenomenon in the therapeutic interchange, we have abandoned the atomistic implications and have begun to regard silence only as a sort of wagnerian *leitmotif* in the drama of psychotherapy.

It is by now well realized that "not all that occurs between therapist and patient is transference and countertransference" (20), and further, that silence is a "happening essentially *between* two people and not inside only one of them" (21). Silence is a production which the patient and the therapist share in authorship. Of necessity, the part played by the therapist contributes *malgré lui* to the many nuances of the therapeutic "atmosphere" (22-28), and has an impact upon the patient and the relationship, sometimes too subtle or too overwhelming to assess.

For instance, one day, in the course of intensive psychotherapy, a middle-aged woman, a chronic schizophrenic, became unusually silent, noticing that I had not turned off the overhead lights in the room as she had requested in a previous session. Fearfully she explained: "You know I don't like overhead lighting . . . I remember I have told you that and yet you seem to forget it every time and leave the lights on . . . (sarcastically) if you have so many patients, why don't you give us a number, write it in a book and remember . . . ?" But again, a few weeks later, the situation repeated itself when the overhead lights were left on. As the hour began, the patient sat intensely tense, preoccupied, and silent. This situation lasted until I became aware that the lights were on. Without a word, I got up and turned them off. Immediately the tension vanished, and the patient showed a warm and understanding smile. With no further comment, the silence was resolved as the patient began speaking on a seemingly unrelated subject.

Another good illustration of the therapist's part in the occurrence of silence took place with another patient, at about her sixth month of therapy, when she became unexpectedly reticent and given to increasingly frequent and prolonged silences. Since her unusual attitude coincided with an effort on my part to stop smoking, I made a guess as to the possible relationship between the two events. The patient then proceeded to explain how to her the fact that I had discontinued smoking meant "disaster . . . for a person who stops smoking soon becomes impatient and nasty . . . ." In spite of this clarification, she remained very cautious and often silent. This situation lasted for several weeks until, about a month later, I resumed smoking and further elucidation became possible. At the sight of my first cigarette, the patient suddenly relaxed, showed a broad smile and greeted the event with a sigh of relief. "Now I am no longer so afraid you will turn nasty and become impatient with me," she said. "To avoid that, I even avoided smoking myself . . . ." She added, "Also, knowing that you were trying to stop smoking, I felt very guilty every time I smoked in front of you . . . but *I couldn't tell you* any of this . . . well, I am very glad you are smoking again!"

Silence is an occurrence in a relationship, and this consideration stands out with particular significance in those situations where silence, far from being an expression of a "negative" mood is, to the contrary, the joyous outcry of a task accomplished, or even the culmination of a progressive step in the therapeutic process. This is the sort of silence that may occur, for instance, as part of the testing out to which the patient subjects the therapist. It is also the sort of silence that may represent an attempt not only to test the therapist's acceptance but in fact to experiment with "one's new wings" and to relish, for instance, the novel experience of dealing with authority figures in a nonsubservient fashion. As a patient clearly expressed it: "I am sure you want me to talk . . . true, you never told me that I must talk, but I am certain that you expect and want me to . . . however, once you also told me that I was the owner of myself . . . I know now that you meant it . . . so . . . (with a triumphant smile not totally carefree) perhaps I will talk tomorrow . . . but I'd rather be silent today!"

Different kinds of silence may be regarded as different sorts of statements in and about a relationship, statements that share the characteristic of being made in the nonverbal mode. Obviously their significance and communicative value are a function of the contextual framework within which they occur. In this regard, it is important to note that not infrequently a particular kind of silence may be followed immediately by another kind of silence, that is to say, *silence may change in kind,* with no noticeable line of demarcation. Although this may constitute a common-place observation, it is curious to note that, to my knowledge, it has not been mentioned in the literature. And yet, this phenomenon of imperceptible change in kind is not, in its essence, unique to silence. In fact, the change that it implies can be noticed in other identified nonverbal situations, such as in crying, particulaly in the crying of an infant. When, for instance, a two- to three-year-old infant is denied an object of his liking, he may begin to cry in frustration and anger; if he is left unattended and no move is made to distract or console him, the infant's cry may soon acquire a different "ring" or quality as it changes in kind from a crying of anger to a crying of painful abandonment. In regard to silence, this change in kind is often observed in psychotherapy.

In the course of psychotherapy with a young schizophrenic woman, it became apparent that often she tended to use silence as a constructive and self-assertive gesture before a therapist whom she construed as authoritarian and exacting. If I remained unresponsive to the gesture and "permissively" allowed its continuance beyond a certain point, her silence would undergo a subtle change in kind and would soon become the vehicle and the expression of her anger and violence. If I again failed to interfere, once more her silence would change in kind, as anger would give place to guilt or ultimately to fear, or both. These three kinds of silence conveyed, therefore, three different messages contextually distinct. Coarsely translated, the first kind of silence said: "I defy you to make me talk . . . I am enjoying the realization that you cannot force me to talk . . . ." The second kind of silence said, "I interpret your silence about my silence as meaning that you have either ignored my message, not caring for me, or are trying to break my silence and take away my triumph . . . either way, *your silence about my silence* makes me angry, very angry at you . . . ." And the third kind of silence said, "I interpret your silence to mean that you are angry at me, probably very angry about my silence . . . I am scared . . . I feel abandoned and helpless . . . I am lost now . . . ." Thus, as the sole expression of a chain of pleasure-anger-fear, her silence changed in kind, subtly and imperceptibly, reflecting the vicissitudes not only of her intrapsychic conflicts but of the patient-therapist relationship.

Parenthetically it may be said that in this sort of situation, the therapist's best opportunity for constructive intervention would occur usually at the point where the first kind of silence (pleasure) would begin to change into the second (anger). At least with this patient it was at such an in-between zone that the simple comment,

"You are enjoying this silence" accompanied and confirmed by a warm voice and unmistakably friendly attitude would suffice to remove the threatening clouds that were beginning to fill the silent atmosphere.

To speak of silence in psychotherapy is to speak not of one, but at least two persons, for silence is an event in a dyad (or polyad) with a significance that cannot be adequately understood outside of the frame of reference within which it occurs. It is apparent that this frame of reference is juxtaposition of several contexts, which includes not only the transferrence but the actual patient-therapist relationship. But what may not be so readily apparent is that psychotherapy, implying factors of much greater import than verbal communication (29, 30), does not necessarily cease when the words stop. Too often the therapist, faced with a silent patient, tends to regard the situation as untenable or even hopeless. And yet, it must be born in mind, that though the silent curtain may fall, therapy can still go on. For in this regard we may recall a bit of popular wisdom and note, paraphrasing, that "silence may speak louder than words." *Res ipsa loquitur.*

Summary

In psychotherapy, silence is to be regarded as an event in the dyad, a production which the patient and the therapist share in authorship. Although the question of the meaning of silence has become obsolete, several different kinds of silence may be distinguished. It is stressed that silence may change in kind, thus in significance, imperceptibly and with no apparent line of demarcation. The importance of this observation is illustrated with clinical material. Silence is to be considered an integral part of relationship, and regarded as neither harmful nor undesirable to therapeutic purpose. For even at the communicational level, as a statement in and about the relationship, silence may be as eloquent as the spoken word.

REFERENCES

1. Plutarch. *Essays*. Little, Brown & Co., Boston, 1881, pp. 342-548.
2. La Rochefoucauld, F. *The Maxims of La Rochefoucauld.* Transl. by L. Kronenberger. Random House, New York, 1959.
3. France, A. *The Wicker-Work Woman, a Chronicle of Our Own Times.* Transl. by M. P. Willcocks. Dodd, Mead & Co., New York, 1923.
4. Shakespeare, W. *Much Ado About Nothing.* Yale University Press, New Haven, 1956, p. 28.

5. ______. *The Tragedy of King Lear.* Yale University Press, New Haven, 1956, p. 12.
6. Shaw, B. Back to Methuselah. *In Selected Plays of Bernard Shaw.* Dodd, Mead & Co., New York, 1949.
7. Freud, S. (1913) The Theme of the Three Caskets. In *Collected Papers,* 4: 244-256, Hogarth Press, London, 1957.
8. ______. (1914) Further Recommendations in the Technique of Psycho-Analysis. Recollection, Repetition and Working Through. In *Collected Papers,* 2: 366-376, Hogarth Press, London, 1957.
9. Meerloo, J. A. M. Free Association, Silence and the Multiple Function of the Speech. *Psychiat. Quart.,* 26: 21, 1952.
10. Abraham, K. First Pregenital Stage of the Libido. In *Selected Papers,* London, Hogarth Press, 1927, pp. 268-230.
11. Ferenczi, S. *Further Contributions to the Theory and Technique of Psycho-Analysis,* Basic Books, New York, 1953.
12. Fliess, R. Silence and Verbalization: A Supplement to the Theory of the "Analytic Rule." *Int. J. Psycho-Anal.,* 30: 21, 1949.
13. Versteeg-Solleveld, C. M. Le Silence. *Folia Psychiat.* 55: 150, 1952.
14. Bergler, E. On the Resistance Situation: The Patient Is Silent. *Psychoanal. Rev.,* 25: 170, 1938.
15. Glover, E. *The Technique of Psyco-Analysis.* International Universities Press, New York, 1955.
16. Greene, A. B. *The Philosophy of Silence.* Richard R. Smith, New York, 1940.
17. Greenson, R. R. On the Silence and Sounds of the Analytic Hour. *J. Amer. Psychoanal. Ass.,* 9: 79, 1961.
18. Kelman, H. Communing and Relating. *Am. J. Psychother.,* 14: 70, 1960.
19. Zeligs, M. A. The Psychology of Silence. *J. Amer. Psychoanal. Ass.,* 9: 7, 1961.
20. Weigert, E. Loneliness and Trust–Basic Factors of Human Existence. *Psychiatry,* 23: 121, 1960.
21. Balint, M. The Three Areas of the Mind; Theoretical Considerations. *Int. J. Psycho-Anal.,* 39: 328, 1958.
22. ______. Changing Therapeutic Aims and Techniques in Psychoanalysis. *Int. J. Psycho-Anal.* 31: 117, 1950.
23. Enelow, A. J. The Silent Patient, *Psychiatry,* 23: 153, 1960.
24. Ferreira, A. J. Psychotherapy with Severely Regressed Schizophrenics. *Psychiat. Quart.,* 33: 664, 1959.
25. Levy, K. Silence in the Analytic Session. *Int. J. Psycho-Anal.,* 39: 50, 1958.
26. Lief, H. I. Silence as Intervention in Psychotherapy. *Am. J. Psychoanal.* 22: 80, 1962.
27. Loewenstein, R. M. Some Remarks on the Role of Speech in Psycho-Analytic Technique. *Int. J. Psycho-Anal.,* 37: 460, 1956.
28. Weisman, A. D. Silence and Psychotherapy. *Psychiatry,* 18: 241, 1955.
29. Ferreira, A. J. The Intimacy Need in Psychotherapy. Presented at the Vth International Congress of Psychotherapy, Vienna, 1961.
30. ______. Loneliness and Psychopathology. *Am. J. Psychoanal.,* 22: 201, 1962.

5

C. E. SCHORER

What Do I Do When the Patient Cries?

Crying is an event of general importance and frequent occurrence in the process of psychotherapy. My more facetious colleagues, when asked to suggest techniques of handling the patient's crying, had little more to offer than that the therapist keep an adequate supply of Kleenex in his office. The present paper is written in the attempt to describe several different ways of responding to crying during the therapeutic interview.

Previous writers have neglected the topic. Ruesch, in *Nonverbal Communication* (1), does not discuss crying, and pictures only the forced crying of pseudobulbar palsy. Greenacre (2), in an article which divides crying into two descriptive types—the shower and the stream—presents examples of each, both symbolic of urination, but the first expressing a partial resignation to, and the second a rejection of, the feminine role. Actually, the examples overlap so much that one could justifiably switch the illustrative cases. LaCombe (3), in a review of one psychoanalytic case, connects weeping with a skin rash and urinary retention, in that both are attempts "to return into mother's skin." These generalizations stem from rather slight evidence, and from a practical point of view the great defect is the failure to say what particular maneuver might be most appropriate for the therapist.

The only recommendations for the therapist of the crying patient are quite general. Both Colby (4) and Wolberg (5) give the advice to handle the patient's crying with reassurance and encouragement.

Reprinted with permission of the author and publisher from the *American Journal of Psychotherapy*, Vol. XVIII, 500-506.

Most wise, but not very specific is an old article by A. N. Foxe (6) on "The Therapeutic Effect of Crying," which states that the appropriate response of the therapist to crying is so delicate and individual a thing as to be beyond the scope of his paper.

To open this topic for more detailed consideration, I would like to sketch four illustrative patterns of therapeutic activity in response to crying.

First, normal crying. This is difficult to illustrate, since a psychiatrist tends to view all visitors to his office as patients. Nevertheless, I will propose the reaction about to be described as normal. A 25-year-old, white American woman, wife of an Iraqi physician, was seen by me at her husband's request to inform her that their application for a permanent visa in the United States had been turned down. He requested that I break the news to her rather than having to do it himself, because he was afraid of her reaction. In obliging him I observed the reaction very much as expected. His wife talked with concern and gravity about their attempt to secure a visa, and when told that it had in fact been denied and that her husband had asked me to tell her the news, she stopped speaking for a moment, became rather flushed and red in the face, and began to cry. She then sobbed quietly for a minute or two, the tears spilling over onto her face and lap, and appeared in great physical distress. After about five minutes there was a certain bitterness in her crying, verbalized spontaneously when she asked, querulously, "Why didn't he tell me himself?" The patient then expressed some more resentment about her husband's reluctance to discuss the situation, and in a few minutes concluded what the best course would be, by saying. "Then there's only one thing to do, and that is to go back"—meaning to go back to Iraq to live. When the husband was subsequently asked to come in and was told that his wife would like to share her feelings more openly with him, he said that I was asking too much; he already was doing as much as he could, and if he had to do this, *he* would have a nervous breakdown.

The situation of this woman was reminiscent of the "acute grief reaction" described by Lindemann in 1954 (7) in connection with the Cocoanut Grove fire, as a specific, rather typical syndrome in which Lindemann emphasized the irregular and almost wild respiration, the intense physical discomfort or distress, and the tendency toward restlessness or physical agitation. Lindemann's recommendations were, of course, that in any acute loss the patient be allowed to work through the grief, give up the old attachment, and form substitutive relations for the lost object, whereby life might be resumed. In a way, the present example is similar, since a sudden revelation was followed almost at once by an appropriate reaction of disappointment; however, it did not lead to marked distortion. The main characteristics of the patient's response was the appropriate sequence of reactions, namely, grief, resentment, and adaptation without any particular intervention by the therapist, except to permit this pattern to take its normal course. Not a word was said to suppress the crying, to show alarm at the possible outcome of restrained weeping, or to interpret its meaning (had I been able to interpret). My sincere attitude, and the attitude I encouraged the patient to take by not intervening, was that an emotional reaction like crying would be normal under these circumstances. She *should* cry, get it over with, and go on with her life.

The second type of crying for the therapist to handle was illustrated by a 24-year-old, married white woman who came for psychotherapy to clear up her marriage problems. She focused on her sexual dissatisfaction and frigidity. Earlier in the marriage she had thought of herself as oversexed, and had been readily aroused by her husband. Because of his premature ejaculation, however, she had repeatedly suffered extreme frustration, ending each time they attempted intercourse by sobbing and feeling terribly upset. Finally, she said, she had steeled herself so that she was no longer aroused by him. The patient's manner in subsequent therapeutic sessions was generally rather cold and detached, although she spoke of emotionally stirring, and indeed traumatic episodes throughout her life. It was as if she had amnesia for the feeling although not for the event. Finally, after about the fifteenth hour, the patient began having great difficulty in speaking. She put on colored glasses, and it was evident from the tone of her voice that she was attempting to keep from breaking into tears. I asked her why she was wearing colored glasses, and she explained that it was so that I would not see her crying. She expanded on this by saying that she never wanted to lose control of herself because it made her vulnerable to ridicule. It was possible to make a connection between her behavior in the interviews (concealing her feelings) and her behavior with her husband in sexual relations (frigidity). The focus in this instance was not on the crying per se, but on the manner in which the patient prevented the therapist from becoming aware of a real demonstration of her feelings. Such a transference and resistance interpretation was invited and made possible by attending to the defensive behavior which accompanied the crying.

The third problem of psychotherapy was the chronic crying of a thirty-eight year old white woman, who had been seen over the years by a large number of professional therapists concerning her domestic problems. I was the third psychiatrist to attempt to treat her with supportive therapy. The meaning of her ubiquitous tears became apparent one day when she described how, as a child, she had found an effective use of tears with her father. All she had to do, she said, was to "turn on the water works," and she could get him to buy her an ice cream cone, or do anything she wanted. A similar strategy worked well with her mother. This was evidence for an interpretation that the crying in the interviews was an attempt to control the therapist and to extract more from him than just understanding her life and her manner of adjusting to it. Here the material related by the patient was used to make an interpretation, and also to make a decision about the future course of therapy. Subsequently, the treatment was directed toward her own manipulativeness rather than toward her grievances. She was encouraged to become independent of these maladaptive techniques.

A final type of therapeutic interaction occurred with a 34-year old woman who had been in treatment two years. Originally she had been hospitalized in an hallucinated state from toxic drug effects, and she also showed mental disorganization resembling a true schizophrenic reaction. Subsequently, the patient frequently went over and over the same material in a quiet way, as though by note. One day, however, when the resident treating her recorded the interview for the purpose of supervision, the patient began to discribe her usual difficulties with husband and mother, but this time interspersed large amounts of anguished crying and sobbing. Since the same material had very often been covered without this display of affect, it was of considerable interest to know why, on this occasion, tears flowed so copiously. The reason became apparent later in the interview and in subsequent sessions when the patient expressed her fear and anger that the recording would be played to the clinic director, with the result that she would not be deemed ill enough to warrant further therapy. It was judged, therefore, that the tears were used both to rebuke the doctor for an anticipated abandonment, and to demonstrate to all concerned her deep need for continuing help. Here, the appropriate activity of the doctor was to observe the unusual affect, and to question why crying was occurring at this juncture. The answer to this question nicely revealed the patient's needs and her strategy for coping with these needs; the answer also paved the way for development of more effective strategies—verbalization, contingency planning, and realistic appreciation of the doctor as a human being with limits to his powers.

These four illustrative types of interaction, while not covering all possibilities, do point up several principles. First, crying appears frequently in psychotherapy and is a potent mode of nonverbal communication. Secondly, in order that the therapist grasp this communication and turn it to use, it is well for him to decide quickly if this is a normal or abnormal response. If this is a normal grief reaction, the therapist would do best to let it run its course.

The therapist, furthermore, may be able to judge the weeping as abnormal if he looks for such clues as a covert manner of crying, habitual crying, and the unexpected appearance of crying in connection with an innocuous topic. If the manner of crying seems unusual, then the manner may be more important to investigate than the grief itself. A question should be directed at once to the patient as to why that particular manner is adopted. Thus, if the patient turns her face away while crying, it may be more important to ask why she turns her face away than why she is crying. If the crying is habitual, the therapist needs to ask the question where this pattern of crying gained its force of habit. The patient then should be encouraged to see that this is an anachronistic maneuver.

If the weeping is unexpected and inexplicable, the therapist had better ask, "Why are you crying?" He certainly needs to recognize that other causes for the crying have to be found, besides the ostensible subject, and it is a matter of tact, whether he should ask this question at once and directly, or not. He may imply that other reasons for crying exist, and that the patient should get them out in the open. He might say, "Tell me what you are thinking about while you are crying." He might say nothing, but eventually, the unexplained cause of crying should be clarified.

Among the complexities I have ignored is the question of physiology. We need to know about the physiologic effects of crying in our patients. Quite apart from "symbolic urethral" expression attached to the act, crying in itself involves conscious tension accumulation and discharge relief. It is well known that many people feel better after a "good cry." It is also known that some people, including most of the male sex in our society, cry very rarely and without the ready discharge benefit other people experience. In treating our patients, we need to understand if crying has a constitutional as well as a psychologic basis–if it is a facile means of discharging anxiety with subsequent relief, inherent in the individual's physiology (8-10). Similarly, from observing several patients who showed a blotchy erythema of the face and neck before and while crying, I would say that a constitutional type exists in which vasodilator and lacrimal responses are synchronized. But I am not at all sure that we should attempt to answer such questions of physiology by investigation during the psychotherapeutic hours.

Finally, the therapist can ask himself what the patient's crying does to him. Has he suddenly offered two or three interpretations or suggestions in a rather wild attempt to be helpful? Has he averted his eyes? Has he sought to ply the patient with a box of Kleenex? Has he found himself tongue-tied? What emotion has this patient aroused, and would that patient have expected, even hoped for this effect?

All these suggestions and questions concerning therapist response to crying are tentative, offered in the hope of opening a topic for more extensive practical consideration. As a result, the next time that the patient cries, or the therapist has a crying patient, one would hope that both would confront this event more effectively and take appropriate steps with greater assurance.

Summary

The crying of the psychotherapy patient requires individualized response. Four examples are given. Normal crying calls for little intervention and may be treated as a healthy phase of adaptation. An unusual and covert manner of crying deserves active inquiry by the therapist about the *manner.* Chronic crying can be handled by the use of an interpretation based on a history of manipulation through crying. Unexpected and abrupt crying should be attended to closely and an explanation sought through appropriate questions. Other questions about the therapy of the crying patient are raised, including consideration of physiology and countertransference.

REFERENCES

1. Ruesch, J., and Kees, W. *Nonverbal Communication.* University of California Press, Berkeley, 1959.
2. Greenacre, P. Pathological Weeping, *Psychoanal. Quart.,* 24: 62, 1945.
3. LaCombe, P. A. A Special Mechanism of Pathological Weeping, *Psychoanal. Quart.,* 27: 246, 1958.
4. Colby, K. *A Primer for Psychotherapists.* Ronald Press, New York, 1951.
5. Wolberg, L. R. *The Technique of Psychotherapy.* Grune & Stratton, New York, 1954.
6. Foxe, A. N. The Therapeutic Effect of Crying, *Medical Record,* 153: 167, 1941.
7. Lindemann, E. Symptomatology and Management of Acute Grief, *Am. J. Psychiat.,* 101: 140, 1944.
8. Montagu, A. Natural Selection and the Origin and Evolution of Weeping in Man. *Science,* 130: 1572, 1959.
9. Brazelton, T. B. Crying in Infancy, *Pediatrics,* 29: 579, 1962.
10. Dunbar, F. *Emotions and Bodily Changes.* Columbia University Press, New York, 1954.

6

W. CLIFFORD M. SCOTT

Patients Who Sleep or Look at the Psychoanalyst During Treatment

Sleeping

For decades psychoanalysts have considered sleep a primary instinct activity. The wish to sleep has been considered to be the contribution of the ego. The aim of the instinct has been "sleep" itself. The object of the instinct has also been described as "the wish to sleep" or "sleep" itself. More has been written about the object of the instinct than about the aim of the instinct. I have not been able to find in the literature the hypothesis which I am putting forward. My hypothesis is: "The total satisfaction of sleep is waking or the act of waking up." Usually the inference is that the aim is sleep—and more sleep.

My observations lead me to conclude that when sleepiness or sleep appears in analysis as a regressive defence, the primary wish to sleep is reactivated since there is in most patients evidence of sleep deprivation. As analysis of such regressive defensive sleep progresses, patients may not only sleep better between interviews but for a time sleep may occur more frequently during interviews. In my opinion the progress of analysis may be speeded rather than retarded by such mixed primary and defensive satisfactions—granted, of course, that all aspects of the activity are brought into analysis. A second conclusion has been that state described as "blankness" and "nothing to talk about," etc. are often defences against sleepiness or sleep. I have concluded that the easiest way to bring the nature of the aim of the impulse into consciousness (of course, in addition to interpretation) is to ask for association to the question "If you slept, how would you like to wake or be wakened?"

Reprinted from the *International Journal of Psychoanalysis*, 1947, Vol. 28, 139.

Behavioristic studies other than of the duration of sleep have not been common. The valuable reports of the effects of experimental sleep deprivation might have been noted more by psychoanalysts who have written about sleep. It was during such studies that delusions of being awake and amnesia of having slept (similar to symptoms frequent in some psychotic depressions) were first described in an experimental setting. Freud in *The Interpretation of Dreams* (1900), *Narcissism* (1914), *Group Psychology* (1921), *New Introductory Lectures* (1923), gradually added to our understanding of sleep as a state of libidinal narcissistic satisfaction. The view that sleep can become a defence against pain was first mentioned by Freud and elaborated by Jones (1923). Jones linked this defence to overcoming the recurrent pain of early extra-uterine tension, but did not advance any hypothesis to account for the gradually decreasing amount of time spent in sleep in infancy. Federn (1932) discussed waking up–chiefly in relation to somnambulism and to depersonalization. Isakower (1938) discussed falling asleep and waking. One example of waking which he gave was the opposite of the descriptions given of "the end of the world" feeling. Waking brought a short-lived cathexis of an omnipotent creative wish–"a world and an ego are created"–like the memory of waking hungry and finding the meal ready. I have observed several similar examples. In the 1942 symposium only Simmel mentioned sleeping during analysis. He was, I think, the first to suggest that waking should be studied in more detail. He described somnambulism as if part of the external world had been internalized, but did not describe somnambulism during interviews where it can be observed and analysed directly. In 1938 at the Paris Congress (published 1947) I described delusional sleep or somnambulism occuring during an interview. I have observed a similar instance since. Lewin (1946) brought a new interest to sleep when he described the "dream-screen" as representing 1) the breast, 2) maximal sleep, 3) the "sleep dream" when sleep is maximal and (tentatively) 4) the mouth-nipple situation. In 1948 Lewin elaborated these observations, but did not follow up the hint of his 1946 paper that a situation, namely, the mouth as well as the breast, is represented in the "dream-screen." Or put in another way–part of what becomes the ego as well as part of what becomes the object may be internalized and may appear in a narcissistic dream. Lewin has come nearest to describing what my experience has been–namely that sleep dreams may be defences against immediate sensory experiences. One such immediate sensory experience might, of course, be that of going to sleep. Recurrently patients express the following sequence of associations–

I have forgotten a dream–
I wish I could remember it–
I have just remembered a dream I had about you–
I feel sleepy–
I want to go to sleep–
If I slept I might dream–
I wish I could remember you but I don't seem able to–
I have just begun to day-dream of you doing something–
I want to look at you, touch you, etc.–
I want you

Such sequences show the relationship between sleep dreams, waking dreams, and immediate sensory experience. Davidson (1945) began to relate sleep to aggression, but did not go so far as to describe an aggressive type of sleep. Jekels (1945) described the slowness of waking as related to waiting in infancy for the satisfaction desired on waking. But waking can be very fast–it can occur in a fraction of a second. The speed at which a patient can fall asleep or wake up has to be clarified. During interviews at least some examples of fast waking and some examples of fast falling asleep are used as defences against memories of a sleep dream or a day dream. Stone (1947) reported a patient who went to sleep as soon as he (Stone) spoke and woke as soon as he stopped speaking. Although such sleep was overdetermined he eventually related it to a conflict between the intrauterine type of sleep and the type of sleep that follows breast feeding.

The following example from my practice will show the type of material on which I have based the hypotheses already mentioned.

The patient was an elderly, energetic, depressed, obsessional man who had come to analysis chiefly for depression associated with rumination about having fallen hopelessly in love thirty years previously. He often went to sleep late at night after spending hours compulsively reading, thinking, or doing crossword puzzles. In the fourth year of analysis a stage was reached when defensive oscillations between early oral and visual interests began to play an important role. He began to have periods of silence whereas previously detailed precise reports had filled interviews. The silences were later described in terms of blankness, but often some emotion was mentioned when the silence was broken. The silences could be understood as defences against communicating annoyance, pleasure, and boredom. His boredom was chiefly related to his wishing me to take action–I was to take the initiative. Recurrently this could be interpreted as similar to the feeding situation in which he had waited blankly and defensively for mother. Only after the blankness, etc., had been interpreted as a defence against sleepiness and sleep, I first realized that he was asleep during a silence when he snored. Previously he had associated to the question "How would you like to wake if you slept?" by stating he would wake as soon as he was spoken to. He appeared to awake immediately when I asked him to try to tell me what had happened, but he was not able to give any memories or associations regarding going to sleep or waking. During later silences I was able to infer that he had been asleep and during sleep had dreamt that he had been awake lying blankly and silently. This inference was possible by my having heard him snore—he couldn't remember sleeping, or waking, or snoring. At other times he relaxed so much that he snored when he was awake. Sometimes after snoring he would say immediately that he had been so relaxed and blank that he had snored, but had not slept. In other interviews we inferred that he had slept and dreamt that he had been awake, blank, relaxed, and that he had snored as sometimes he told me he had snored when I had not heard him. Evidence accumulated regarding the unconscious conflict about going to sleep and waking up. He remained unconscious of any conflict about talking of the sensations, memories, images, etc., when he was very sleepy—he went to sleep instead. He was also either passive with regard to waking up (he woke immediately when I spoke) or unconscious of waking up. When I interpreted that the psycho-analytic situation was so allied to his feelings of the feeding situation that he was not separating them, he became conscious of the fact that he could neither have a phantasy nor a memory of the situation he was in (he had no sensations of his body on the couch when he became blank)—he began to realize how very blank the blankness had been. He became more silent and slept more. Once after mentioning that one way of dealing with weaning was to become a woman and of how much more like a child he felt with a new female friend, he became silent and after three or four minutes snored. After thirty minutes he was asked to try to talk of how he wanted to sleep or wake—he said "I was hovering between sleeping and waking up—it was different from the other times—I wonder if the level was fluctuating—or did I dream I was awake—it didn't seem that I was awake—did I snore—I had the impression that I had it within my power to think of something—but I didn't want to think of anything—the position here was like in water or in a liquid—I could be on the surface—or in it to various depths." These associations were interpretated as referring to a defensive oscillation between wishing to be conscious of his mother—(he had said—"I could think of something") or to be conscious of me (he had said "As soon as you spoke I was instantly attentive"). I connected his statement of "thinking about something" and "feeling as if in a liquid" with the early feeling of both having taken his mother into him and of his having gone into his mother. I connected his talk of thinking (his thoughts are very much inside) and his talk of feeling (feelings to him are mostly something other people have) with the split he had made between thinking and feeling—between the mouth and the nipple. The first fifteen minutes of the next interview dealt (1) with the access of energy he had felt since the previous day; (2) with a dream he had forgotten which he felt was connected with his wishes to be a woman or to be bisexual and (3) with his desires to be rid of having so much satisfaction from intellectual activity. On this note he became silent. After fifteen minutes he said in a sleepy voice "Something to do with a balloon—I didn't use it—like my dream last night"—after ten minutes' further silence he suddenly said "Did you say—no—no, you couldn't—I must have been dreaming." His associations were to his hiding breast memories behind his intellect—to wondering whether thinking is like a cow ruminating—to anger at not being able to enjoy pleasure in psychoanalysis—to anger at my not giving him the pleasure he would have liked his mother to have given him—to his wanting me to make use of his productions as he would have liked his mother to have appreciated his sucking.

In these examples I think I have given enough material to show

how "working through" may mean dealing with many periods of silence, sleepiness, and the sleep before the patient approaches consciousness of the primary sleep wish and wake wish.

Looking

Interest in sleep and its connection with oral satisfaction led me to what I think may be new observations connecting oral motor sensations and oral touches with sounds and sights, skin sensations, etc. and with feelings of movements which spread to the stomach, the bladder, the bowels, etc. Just as we lack descriptions of primary waking (if there is such a state) we lack descriptions of the early type of waking before looking or waking in order to see. We know much about the later derivatives of looking and sleeping (e.g. the visual sleep dream) but little about the origins of the connection between looking and waking.

Patients show unconscious desires to look; impulsive acts of looking; conscious wishes to look; phantasies of what the psychoanalyst will look like if they look and deliberate acts of looking and descriptions of what is seen.

During psychoanalysis of children looking recurrently comes into interviews, but usually not until adolescence does the problem arise of how psychoanalysis can be carried on most efficently as far as the ocular relationship between analyst and patient is concerned.

When a patient looks away, or doesn't like being looked at, or wants to hide his facial expression, or doesn't want to be concerned any more about what his face looks like, etc., we are usually up against anxieties about the body surface on the one hand and the inner situation on the other. With adolescents I have found defensive oscillations between looking at and looking away from the analyst continue more or less until the end of treatment. With adolescents one sees more clearly the relationship between the looking that usually occurs at the beginning and at the end of the interviews and the recurrent desires to look or actual looking during the interviews. Adolescent looking can usually be quickly connected with anxieties about acting out other desires, touching, for instance. I have found that, if the defences (and some are, of course, the beginnings of ego-syntonic defences) and both the substitute and primary impulses are analysed, there may be for a time more looking but also more progress.

With adults the situation is different. Here I should describe my couch. It is flat, well-sprung, 6¾ x 3 feet, has no back, and is not against a wall. Patients use one, two or no pillows, a pillow cover, and a rug beneath their feet. I sit behind the couch at one end. The cushions are on the couch at the beginning of an interview. In other words, the position of the pillows suggests a way for the patient to lie. Nevertheless the shape and position of the couch do not cramp movements as some psycho-analytic couches do. Some patients start analysis with "Of course, you don't like to be looked at, do you–Freud didn't like it, did he?" But there are also naive patients who have never heard of Freud and flop down, elbows on the pillow, chin cupped in palms with a "now what" expression. Patients may lie on their back or stomach, they may lie on their right or their left sides, or they may wish to lie with their head at the opposite end of the couch, but each movement, position, or wish can furnish material for furthering the analysis.

The variations between such wishes, postures or movements can be discussed under the headings of reality, symbolism and transference.

The Reality Problem.

A patient may say "Why shouldn't I look–the cat can look at the Queen," etc. This attitude may persist until its implications in the situation have been interpreted and worked through. Often the patient looks to hide defences against remembering or anticipating. The patient may use looking in order to avoid the psychoanalytic rule, namely, verbalization of what is conscious. Each look or ocular change is accompanied by a change in consciousness unless, of course, the patient is unconscious of having looked or of having seen anything. One problem with children and adults, whether neurotic, psychotic, defective, or normal is to discover how ocular activity can hinder or help the progress of analysis.

Symbolism.

There is always overdetermination in the act of looking. This was illustrated by a patient who always looked when she said she couldn't eat. She had to look in order to see that she hadn't eaten. Looking can symbolize functions, such as eating or vomiting. Looking can symbolize a mechanism–introjection or projection. Interpreting acts of looking may lead to the first insight the patient develops regarding a new zonal activity or a new mechanism. A patient may wish he had an eye somewhere else and his eyes may move. The eye may be symbolic of some other organ. Much displaced material may be worked through first in terms of ocular memories, fantasies, or acts before it is worked through in its primary terms.

Transference.

Discrepancies between the memory or anticipatory image of the analyst and the sensation of the analyst give material for transference interpretation and often stimulate counter-transference with its stimulus to self–anlysis. The patient may say one looks dead, scornful, tired, relaxed, nice, etc., and such remarks may be repeated in a persevering manner–in other words, the patient may keep observing, hoping the expression will change. Usually such perseveration is a defence against looking away or closing the eyes to see more clearly what the wish is. Looking at a minute detail of facial expression will often stimulate the wish or act as a defence against the wish to analyze the analyst. Mutual looking by the patient and analyst is not as incompatible as is mutual talking at the same time. Mutual looking in this way is often related to kissing or fighting or other acts that can be mutual. Consciousness of the eye plus the mouth often becomes the substitute for that which was earlier primarily entirely perceived as oral. Sometimes a patient may watch the movements of the analyst's lips and tongue (keeping his mouth meanwhile wide open) and he may not hear what was said. Such behavior gives the opportunity of interpreting regression to the time of lack of discrimination between noise made by the mother and noise made by the rest of the world and to the time of lack of discrimination of the eye as an organ of sight. At such times cathexis of the open eyes and open mouth appear to be equally shared.

Just as technique developed in adult psychoanalysis paved the way for child analysis, so also aspects of technique brought into adult analysis from child analysis may create a situation in which oscillations between the regression and progression can occur more rapidly, allowing little bits of experience to be worked through at a time. In child analysis body movements are allowed expression, made use of in interpretation, and furnish one of the ways we observe ego development during analysis. In adult analysis greater use of movement[1] – including eye movements–may increase the speed and depth of analysis. By such experiments we may become able to bring into adult analysis the implications of earlier and earlier problems, and perhaps we may learn how to prevent the occasional long-term regressions which may occur during psychoanalytic treatment and which make further analysis difficult.

Summary

If more attention is paid to defences against sleeping and looking as well as to their substitute and primary instinctive aspects, and increased amount of sleeping and looking may enter the analytic situation. Such a development may furnish new material to be used

1. Did time permit, detailed reference should be made to the recent work of Hoffer regarding hand movements and to Felix Deutsch and Gostynski regarding general body movement.

in interpretations and may speed rather than retard the progress of the analysis.

REFERENCES

1. Davidson, C. (1945). *Psychoanal. Quart.*, 14, 478.
2. Federn, P. (1932). *Psychoanal. Quart.*, 1, 511.
3. Freud, S. (1900). *Interpretation of Dreams*. London: Allen and Unwin.
   _______ (1914). "On Narcissism." *Collected Papers*, Vol. 4. London: Hogarth Press.
   _______ (1921). *Group Psychology and the Analysis of the Ego*. London: Hogarth Press.
   _______ (1923). *New Introductory Lectures on Psycho-Analysis*. London: Hogarth Press.
4. Isakower, O. (1936). (Trans. 1938) *Int. J. Psycho-Anal.*, 19, 331.
5. Jekels, L. (1945). *Psychoanal. Quart.*, 14, 169.
6. Jones, E. (1923). *Papers on Psycho-Analysis.* 3rd Edition. Introduction. London: Bailliere, Tindall & Cox.
7. Lewin, B. D. (1946). *Psychoanal. Quart.*, 15, 419.
   _______ (1948). *Int. J. Psycho-Anal.*, 29, 224.
8. Scott, W. C. M. (1947). *Int. J. Psycho-Anal.*, 28, 139.
9. Simmel, E. (1942). *Int. J. Psycho-Anal.*, 23, 65.
10. Stone, L. (1947). *Int. J. Psycho-Anal.*, 28, 18.

7

MELVIN L. SELZER

The Use of First Names in Psychotherapy

The success of psychotherapy may be jeopardized by an infinite variety of factors. These are usually introduced by the patient but may on occasion be the unconscious contribution of the psychotherapist. Inasmuch as we are concerned with the welfare of our patients, it is vitally important that we be frequently reminded that *everything* we do as psychoterapists should be for the benefit of the patient. Anything the therapist does that fails to meet this criterion has no place in the therapeutic setting.

Addressing adult patients by their first names has become a rather common practice–a practice that may well exert considerable influence on the course of psychotherapy. If the practice of addressing adult patients by their first names does not specifically benefit the patient, and indeed may be injurious to the goals of psychotherapy, the conscientious therapist will agree to the elimination of this practice.

An effort will be made to shed some light on this phenomenon, the possible reasons for it, and its potential effect on both patient and therapist.

The Need to Feel Superior

One possible reason for addressing patients by their first names may be the anxiety engendered in the insecure therapist when he fears his patient may be more intelligent, more successful, or better endowed in some way than he. In addressing patients by their first

Reprinted from the *Archives of General Psychiatry*, 1960, Vol. 3, 215-218.

names, these psychiatrists may unconsciously be attempting to reduce their patients to subordinate and hence less threatening figures. Perhaps an example of this mechanism from a different, although equally familiar, segment of the psychiatric scene will help to emphasize this point.

In many state mental hospitals, one quickly becomes aware of the fact that attendants will address patients by their first names although insisting that they be addressed in a more formal manner (i.e., Mrs., Mr., etc.). Attendant personnel are often underpaid and not infrequently drawn from deprived segments of the population. Added to this is their relatively low status in the hospital hierarchy and an almost total unawareness of their potentially useful role in the rehabilitation of patients.

In this setting one can perceive the attendant's need to establish himself as being superior to the patient group and to achieve some gratification from these feelings of superiority. One way to implement this sense of superiority or authority is to address patients by their first names, regardless of their age, previous achievements, or mental status, while making it quite clear that hospital personnel must be addressed in a more dignified manner.

Although one can readily comprehend (but not condone) a hospital attendant's motives for insisting on calling patients in his care by their first names, the psychotherapist's motives for doing so may be more obscure.

Fromm-Reichmann (1) has cautioned against psychiatrists "assuming an attitude of personal, irrational authority instead of . . . conducting therapy in a spirit of collaborative guidance. Only a self-respecting psychiatrist can respect his patients and meet them on a basis of mutual human equality."

Even competent psychiatrists often harbor feelings of guilt because they are not personally and professionally perfect. They may attempt to compensate for their real or fancied deficiencies by attempting to reduce patients to a level where they feel comfortable enough to deal with them. If the competent therapist can accept the idea that he is not supposed to be perfect, there would be less need to place the patient on a lower plane.

Minimizing the Patient's Illness

Thus far I have dealt with the psychiatrist's insecurity impelling him to "minimize" the patient. However, the therapist's uncertainty regarding his competence to cope with psychopathology may also create a need for him to minimize the patient's *illness*. It is as if the therapist unconsciously reasons: "If there is not too much wrong with the patient, then even I can help him." For example, a therapist whose training or position is such that he feels he can only deal with minor adjustment problems may tend to underdiagnose his patients, thus perceiving psychoses as neuroses and neuroses as adjustment problems (2).

One way to minimize the patient's illness is to regard it as a temporary adolescent-like difficulty (2), implementing this by addressing the patient as one would a child: by given name. The implication is: "You are still a child—your problems couldn't be serious." Fromm-Reichmann has stated, "Patients feel encouraged if the psychiatrist realizes the severity of their difficulties and does not minimize them." (1) This is an important therapeutic principle regardless of the etilolgy or severity of a patient's illness.

Avoiding Therapeutic Commitment

There is another possible reason for the "helpless" therapist addressing patients by their first names. In so doing, he may unknowingly be seeking to convert the interviews into semisocial occasions, thus relieving himself of the uncomfortable obligation of helping the patient.

The above mechanism was suggested by a recent conversation with a respected colleague. When apprised of the subject of this paper, he confessed that he had but one patient whom he addressed by first name. This was a young woman who suffered from no specific psychiatric disorder. She had come to him because her husband had recently been institutionalized for a psychotic breakdown, her father was dying a lingering death from a metastatic carcinoma, and she was on the verge of being asked to leave college because of academic deficiencies.

Obviously the psychiatrist could not materially alter his patient's painful situation. As suggested above, he may have felt that the maintenance of a formal doctor-patient relationship would constitute a promise to the patient that he could not fulfill. The spontaneous decision to use the patient's first name was intended to avoid commitment in a situation which he felt was beyond his immediate professional scope.

In giving interviews a casual air by using the patient's first name, the psychiatrist may in effect be indicating that he and the patient are merely chatting. He cannot offer the patient much effective help. Thus he seeks to avoid responsibility (and perhaps feelings of guilt) in the event that the patient fails to obtain a beneficial result from the time spent with him. At this point we must ask if this approach is good for the patient? The troubled patient may soon sense that the therapist is no longer professionally committed and is in effect merely passing the time of day. Even the potentially supportive and reassuring effect the therapy could afford the patient is thereupon nullified. The patient is left with his or her original problems plus the haunting realization that even the therapist cannot, or is not trying to help.

"Friendship"

A number of therapists will use a patient's first name as a friendly gesture that they hope will make it easier for the patient to relate to them. Since one addresses friends by their first names, this usage implies an offer of friendship. This technique deserves careful scrutiny. A patient who is offered friendship may feel a need to retain that friendship. (This is particularly so of psychiatric patients who frequently have had lifelong difficulty with object relationships.) To retain the therapist's friendship, the patient may feel constrained to forego discussing aspects of his personality that he feels would offend or alienate the therapist. (This is not surprising inasmuch as friendships are not based on total frankness, but on mutual consideration and affection.)

A statement made by a patient regarding his previous therapist might serve to illustrate the above point. "I felt like she was a mother to me–she was such a motherly person. So I began to lie to her about the things I was doing. You see, I didn't want to disappoint her. After a while I saw it was silly to go there and tell lies, and I quit going."

A psychotherapeutic relationship based on friendship may meet with initial success but can ultimately hinder the patient's freedom to express himself. Paradoxically, a professional approach to the patient makes it easier for the patient to ultimately reveal those things that trouble him most. At this point it becomes necessary to ponder why the therapist may feel a need to appear "friendly." Patients in psychotherapy not infrequently vent a great deal of hostile feeling on the therapist. This is not always easy to take, and the therapist may have difficulty handling his own counterhostility and anxiety under these circumstances. The therapist may anticipate this by trying to be friendly in an attempt to avert and avoid the patient's hostility. In the same vein, the "friendly first name approach" may be the therapist's reaction formation against his own unconsciously anticipated feelings about the inevitable appearance of hostility in his patients.

What has been said about hostility, and counterhostility, can also be said about anxiety. Therapists who have difficulty handling their own anxiety may be unable to comfortably face an anxious patient. They may attempt to reassure the patient by using their first names in an effort to appear "friendly" so that the patient will not become more anxious. However, any premature attempt to reassure a patient that is not based on an understanding of the patient's problems is doomed to failure. In fact, it may well have the opposite effect since the patient will realize that the therapist does not have enough information to realistically reassure him and is in fact reassuring himself (1).

The Danger of Regression

The patient appeals to the psychiatrist for help with emotional problems usually involving some degree of anxiety. Anxiety, itself a regressive phenomenon, not infrequently produces a tendency to further regression to an earlier level in an attempt to recapture the real or fancied comfort of the earlier period. Initially the patient may be relieved to have his regressive tendencies encouraged by a child-parent relationship with the therapist. Ultimately, however, the patient may realize that this approach has rendered him less capable of facing future difficulties alone. If the therapist first cultivates the patient's dependence, it pushes the patient into a greater state of dependence at the expense of working toward greater maturity and ability to use his own judgment. The patient's initial relief may turn to resentment at what he perceives to be the therapist's interference with his tendency toward and wish for growth and independence, since these are almost invariably among the goals which the patients seek in coming for psychiatric help (1).

Summary and Conclusion

The practice of addressing adult patients in psychotherapy by their first names has been discussed. A number of speculative reasons for this phenomenon have been advanced. These include the need to feel superior to the patient, the need to minimize the patient's illness, and the tendency to avoid therapeutic commitment. In addition, the limitations of the "friendship" approach and the danger of encouraging regression were pointed out. The possible deleterious effects of this practice on the self-esteem of the patient and on the psychotherapeutic relationship have been emphasized.

Any practice that may diminish the patient's self-respect carries with it the additional hazard of creating unrealistic feelings of superiority in the therapist. Marmor (4) has characterized grandiosity in the therapist as an ego defense against anxiety. He points out that as a consequence of both realistic factors and the transference phenomenon it is all too easy for the therapist to perceive himself as a superman. Any technique that promotes grandiosity in the therapist may not only undermine the therapeutic relationship but will also interfere with the constant re-examination of one's therapeutic methods, goals, and motives so necessary for continued professional growth and clinical effectiveness.

Although it is conceivable that the use of an adult patient's first name may be warranted in some instances, the psychotherapist should first ascertain that he has an unequivocally valid reason for addressing the patient in this manner.

REFERENCES

1. Fromm-Reichmann, F.: Principles of Intensive Psychotherapy, Chicago, University of Chicago Press, 1950.
2. Selzer, M.: The Happy College Student Myth: Psychiatric Implications, A.M.A. Arch. Gen. Psychiat. 2:131 (Feb.) 1960.
3. Arieti, S.: Interpretation of Schizophrenia, New York, Robert Brunner, Inc., 1955, p. 54.
4. Marmor, J.: The Feeling of Superiority: An Occupational Hazard in the Practice of Psychotherapy, Am. J. Psychiat. 110:370 (Nov.) 1953.

8

HELEN STEIN

The Gift in Therapy

Yet gifts should prove their use
I own the past profuse
Of power each side, perfection every turn:
Eyes, ears, took in their dole
Brain treasured up the whole,
Should not the heart beat once,
"How good to live and learn."
–*Rabbi Ben Ezra* by Robert Browning

Introduction

Giving and receiving gifts has always been an elemental and universal form of human interchange. The paucity of literature on the meaning of gifts in therapy is therefore surprising and suggestive of a hidden problem regarding the gift, the giver, and the recipient (1). One is reminded of Virgil's saying in the *Anead* "I fear gifts and the bearers of gifts"; more familiarly, "Beware of Greeks bearing gifts." Psychotherapy, which nourishes a close and extended relationship under trained scrutiny, offers a fertile field for the study of the psychology of giving, taking, and receiving, and the underlying fantasies.

In the available psychiatric literature we find no definitive attitude toward gifts: "As a general rule an analyst should not accept gifts, but he should also know when to make an exception. When a patient who has great difficulty in giving anything is able, in the course of treatment, to make the analyst a small present, it would be a serious mistake not to accept the gift" (2).

The little gift which is sent impulsively should be graciously received, Lorand comments.

Reprinted with permission of the author and publisher from the *American Journal of Psychotherapy*, Vol. XIX (1965), 480-486.

> However, the patient's actions must be analyzed as thoroughly as possible, and he should be brought to realize that, although it is a gesture of affection or an attempt at bribery, at the same time . . . . he also harbors feelings of hostility and aggression towards the analyst. . . . No matter how satisfactorily the analyst can rationalize to himself his acceptance of an expensive gift, it is still due to deep, unconscious problems concerning giving and taking which were not clarified and successfully worked out in his own analysis (3).

Acceptance of a gift offers both gratification and reassurance, as pointed out by Glover:

> It seems that analysts can take a more definite stand for or against "reassurance" so long as these problems are discussed solely in terms of verbal interpretation and verbal reassurance. Some of those who were against verbal reassurance [in answers to a questionnaire] . . . were, nevertheless, not against accepting small gifts. . . . It is reassuring to the patient (4).

Derivation of Words for "Gifts"

The gift in therapy may be a valuable parameter of human communication and a symbolic expression of human needs on various levels, a reflection of the complexity of human functioning.

The word "gift" itself is derived from Middle English, from Old Norse, and from Old English, where the root is *giefans.* Latin distinguishes the gift which signifies a special talent from gift as *donum* and gift as *praemium,* which has the connotation of bribe. The various connotations of gifts are more sharply distinguished in the Spanish language, *don* being one obligation in return for another, *favor* meaning support and protection, *regalo* a gift to give pleasure, and *oblacion* a sacrificial offering. The German distinguishes between two kinds of giving, *schenken* and *geben.* Connotations of *Gabe* are "to forgive"–*vergeben*–from Old High German and "tongue" from Biblical German. The root words of gift as *Geschenk* come from Old High German and mean "to pour out." *Schenk* is a cup bearer, *Schenke* is an inn, and *Schenkel* is the thigh or femur. One is reminded of the Biblical displacement of the phallus to the thigh. There is also the expression for having children–*Kinder schenken.* Abraham, in his *Collected Papers,* points out that, in certain districts of Germany, the act of suckling a child is called *schenken,* to give or to pour (5).

Actually in German the word *Gift* signifies poison (by common usage). The first indication of an ambivalence about gifts arises here in the study of word derivations. The English word "*dose*" as something given comes from the Latin *dosis,* whereas the Greek root signifies a dose of poison. In 1848 the German scholar Karl Ludwig Grimm published a definitive study of the two German words, in a treatise entitled "Uber Schenken und Geben" (6). He pointed out that, in the Sanskrit, dadâmi is "gift," uddâna means "tying" or "binding," and nidana is "string." Moreover, if the Greek letters n and w are transposed into their Sanskrit equivalent—â—the Greek words for "I give" and "I bind" are identical. Here we have the gift—sacrifice to the gods—bound down to symbolize that the gods were bound in return.

Cultural History of Gifts

Marcel Mauss (7), in his posthumous book on gifts in archaic societies, came to this conclusion: "Although the form usually taken is that of the gift, generously offered, the accompanying behavior is based on obligation and economic self-interest." Exchanges are not exclusively of goods, wealth, and property but also of courtesies, entertainments, military assistance, dances and feasts, rituals, women, and children, always with counter-presentations.

The American Indians have a type of obligatory gift giving which binds the group both to give and to receive. In Samoa there are contractual gifts at childbirth, circumcision, sickness, girls' puberty, funerals, and trade agreements. Gifts must be returned. The Samoan child is regarded as a piece of property and is regularly given to the maternal uncle. For the Maori the gift has a spirit, *hau,* which is considered a part of the giver. To return the gift gives the recipient power over the original giver; to keep the gift becomes dangerous. The magic expectations of the giver are not to be minimized. The gift is always given in some context.

The Andaman Islanders off the Australian Coast have an abundant economy and use gift giving competitively to see who can give the most. The Melanesians, on the other hand, sometimes destroy all their own property so that they may neither give nor receive. The Trobrianders, made famous by Malinowski, have symbolic gifts. Their currency is jewelry, armshells and rings being female symbols and necklaces male symbols. The gift binds the recipient to a return gift of a tooth. The Brahmins and the Chinese considered gifts obligatory and actually a part of the body of the giver.

In the evolution of human society, we come to gifts as sacrifice, with the same contexts as in archaic societies (8). From food as a plea for sustenance, to animal sacrifice, to the full explosion of murder and cannibalism in human sacrifice, the gamut of need, anger, and destruction has a worldwide distribution. E. B. Tylor regarded the sacrifice as a gift made to the gods in the spirit of self-abnegation implying, If I deprive myself my parent will aid me. (9) In the totemic meal the theme of atonement for the acting out of hostile impulses, originally pointed out by W. Robertson Smith in his *Religion of the Semites* is masterfully developed by Freud in *Totem and Taboo* (10). The feast during funeral celebrations or prior to days of fasting is another variant of the totemic meal of oral incorporation, guilt, and atonement. One wonders whether the act of suicide may not be a murder, an atonement, and the gift of the self to the persecutory introjected image.

Symbolism of Gifts in Therapy

Thus we have a communion with the past in the universality, symbolism, and archaism of gifts. The patient too is a living link to a past. He has his history and his symbolism and his development. And he may be the bearer of gifts. Oral needs emerge clearly in the need to be fed when a patient brings a gift of food. It is a desire for abundant nourishment and a talisman to guard against one's greed of wishing to devour all.

> I had a patient who had been hospitalized for 20 years; each time she came into my office she felt compelled to bring me food or drink. After I came to know her better, I asked her why she always brought me food. She said that no doctor ever bothered to talk to her anymore because she had been hospitalized for so many years. She remembered that her mother, who had smothered her with food, had then ridiculed her for being fat. The hunger was unmistakable under the anger, and the need to return the food and reverse the feeding was there. The food was always wrapped in a beautiful container in the spirit of a gift.

> Another patient, a lady with diabetes and arthritis, brought an ugly brown piece of sculpture each time she came. She rebelled against her illness, her ugliness. She made my office ugly. But she offered herself, even as ugly and misshapen. Would I accept what she had to give? Could I make her whole and beautiful?

The baby takes his food, smiles, and learns sphincter control. All he has to give at first is of bodily origin. Later he may make or buy things.

Karl Abraham pointed out that the expectations of childhood are often seen in terms of gifts. "In the eyes of the child a proof of love is almost the same thing as a *gift*. The first proof of love which creates a lasting impression . . . is being suckled. . . . Within certain limits the child repays its mother's 'gift' in return." The little boy is afraid that his penis may be detached from his body in the same way as his feces are. The little girl expects the missing penis to be given her as a gift, first from her mother and then later from her father. That being impossible, she hopes to get a child (5, pp. 342-343).

The bodily derivation of gifts has been known to anthropologists, but it was Freud who clearly formulated the unconscious equation gift=feces=money=baby=penis; and breasts=penis. "Those who question this derivation of gifts should consider their experience of psychoanalytic treatment, study the gifts they receive as doctors from their patients, and watch the storms of transference which a gift from them can rouse in their patients" (11).

The patient who presents the doctor with a plant may wish to remain rooted in the office. She may wish to be nourished, helped to grow, handled with care. She may magically expect the gift returned in terms of breast, penis, or child reflecting her developmental level. She is beautifying your office and may wish to be herself made more beautiful. Flowers are commonly used in courtship, at weddings, births, and funerals.

I remember well a patient who was literally terrified of the plants in my office. She said they reminded her of funerals. She was so terrified of her death wishes against her father, and of the fact that her mother was already dead, that she was afraid to go to sleep. She would keep the light on all night for fear of being killed in retaliation. Another patient, who particularly liked to give flowers and wear flowered dresses and pins, had defloration fears and fantasies. A present of red roses enabled her to recall from the repressed her self-defloration at the age of four when she scratched herself intensely during a severe attack of chicken pox.

A schizophrenic girl, when faced by the prospect of her first separation from me, impulsively picked up a man and had intercourse with him, without the use of contraceptives. She then signed herself back into the hospital in a panic about becoming pregnant. She was expressing the need for me to take care of her and, more urgently, her baby. Substituting me for a baby, she could carry me around within her body and show her anger at me for leaving and contempt for me as a woman. The only gift I could not give her was a baby. She remained in the hospital for the month I was away and could not be convinced that she was not pregnant until I returned. Interestingly enough, she expressed a fear of giving me a present although she often wished to do so. And she had fantasies about bisexual figures, an expression of the wish to have and the fear of having the phallic mother with the "extra gift."

Gifts as a Form of Recollection

If we regard the gift as a fragment of communication, it plays in the analysis an intermediate role between the dream fragment and a form of acting out. The manifest content then has relevance to the present and the latent content has relevance to the past. It is a form of recollection, and discloses what the dream illustrates. The gift may substitute a part for the whole; it may condense several meanings; it may express infantile desires, hatreds, revenge, and death wishes. It may be a memory of crucial events of birth, death, seduction, marriage, trauma, primal scenes, and mourning rites. It courses over the full gamut of the analytic work. In terms of acting out, the gift substitutes the magic of action for verbal recollection; it dramatizes; it pleases the eye; it is an escape from a severe superego; it reproduces the feeding and excreting at the will of the patient, and relieves an intolerable anxiety (12).

> A gift of yellow roses aided a patient in the recollection of having worn a yellow dress as a child and being slapped the only time in her life by her father for telling him that she looked pregnant in the yellow dress. The anger was repressed along with the death wishes, and later the yellow dress was used to seduce a playmate. Anger, love, guilt, seduction, and a reversal of roles were here the content of a gift of yellow roses from a woman patient to a male therapist.

Gifts as Defense

Gifts then serve a defensive function in the sense of being a talisman against both hostile and erotic wishes. The gift expresses, substitutes, and wards off these wishes. Simultaneously it becomes a reparation for destructive fantasies against loved objects. The giver seeks to bind the therapist to himself for both nourishment and protection. Klein (13), emphasizing pregenital aggression and guilt, refers to symbolic reparation for wishes to rob and incorporate the mother's breast and the father's penis. Lewinsky (14) speaks of five types of giving: 1) propitiary–to assure welcome as the person feels himself unwanted; 2) deceptive–to assuage anger and coerce the recipient into kindness; 3) assertive–to proclaim the ability to give and to deny hoarding and greed; 4) substitutive–to offer a gift to be "devoured" instead of the patient; and 5) fetishistic–as protection or talisman against fear of anger and sexuality which has become identified with murder and rape. Acceptance of the gift proves the goodness of the giver, makes him welcome and protects, while it communicates and gratifies as well. If it is to aid in the mastery of anxiety, the giving of gifts should not be interpreted or curtailed too soon.

Gifts as a Form of Magic Action

It becomes important to know the patient and the particular fantasy underlying the gift at the time it is being given.

> One of my patients, who worked outside but lived in the hospital, came in one day to say goodbye and tell me she was leaving. As a parting gift she gave me her paycheck, which she usually sent to her mother and small son. She was dressed in black. I could not escape the feeling that she intended to commit suicide; and when I confronted her with this feeling, she was overwhelmed and confirmed my judgment. She was in a state of stupor and excitement for several weeks as reparation for her intense guilt. She had wished permission to kill herself, her mother, her son, and her lover. She was unable to grieve and mourn.
>
> A way of mourning was accessible to another patient who would leave a

gift with a calling card in the waiting room without seeing the therapist. This was a reenactment of visiting the grave of her father and the mourning, which was curtailed both by intensity of grief and unresolved guilt.

The work of repetition, recollection, and working through is the real work of therapy (15). It encompasses the oral pleasures and trauma of weaning, the anal pleasures of retaining and giving, the phallic stage of excitement, castration fears, penis envy, object-loss and grief and symbolic restitution. Finally a genital form of complete giving with consideration for the real needs of the recipient emerges.

One must sense the "right time" for an interpretation through an awareness of the fantasy life and the current needs of the patient. The therapist must have a clear knowledge of his own equilibrium between give and take. It is far easier to refuse a gift; but one must know how and when to accept a gift. The "transference love," although its roots are in infantile life, is powerful and genuine indeed. "There is no love that does not reproduce infantile prototypes," Freud wrote. "One has no right to dispute the 'genuine' nature of the love which makes its appearance in the course of analytic treatment" (16). The love embodied in the gift outlives the giver, affirms his life drive, and adds a sense of beauty to the endurance of life.

Summary

Gifts presented during therapy are a special form of communication, having roots in unconscious fantasy. The patient symbolically gives the therapist a gift on an oral, anal, phallic, or genital level and wishes to bind the therapist to a gift in return. Gifts serve as a defense against both hostile and erotic impulses. They are a form of "magic action," intermediate between dreaming and acting out. They may also conceal a repressed traumatic memory. The proper interpretation of a gift may mark a crucial turning point in therapy.

The author would like to thank George J. Train, M.D. for his kindness and inspiration with regard to this study.

REFERENCES

1. Meerloo, J. A. Santa Claus and The Psychology of Giving. *Am. Practitioner,* 11-12, 1031-1035, 1960.
2. Van der Walls, H. G. In Menninger K., *Theory of Psychoanalytic Technique,* Basic Books, New York, 1958, p. 40.
3. Lorand S. *Technique of Psychoanalytic Therapy.* International Universities Press, New York, 1946, pp. 220-222.
4. Glover, E. *Technique of Psychoanalysis.* International Universities Press, New York, 1955, pp. 319-320.
5. Abraham, K. *Collected Papers.* Hogarth Press, London, 1949, p. 342.
6. Grimm, K. L. J. *Uber Schenken und Geben. Preussische Academie der Wissenschaften,* Berlin, October 26, 1848.
7. Mauss, M. *Gifts–Forms and Functions of Exchange in Archaic Societies.* Cohen & West, London, 1954.
8. Money-Kyrle, R. *The Meaning of Sacrifice.* Hogarth Press, London, 1929.
9. Kardiner, A. *The Individual and his Society.* Columbia University Press, New York, 1955, p. 304.
10. Freud, S. *Totem and Taboo.* W. W. Norton, New York, 1962.
11. Freud, S. Transformation of the Instincts. In *Collected Papers,* Vol. 2, Basic Books, New York, 1959.
12. Greenacre, P. General Problems of Acting Out. In *Trauma, Growth and Personality.* W. W. Norton, New York, 1952, pp. 224-236.
13. Klein, M. and Riviere, J. *Love, Hate and Reparation.* Hogarth Press, London, 1937.
14. Lewinsky, H. Pathological Generosity. *Int. J. Psycho-Anal.* 32:185, 1959.
15. Freud, S. Repetition, Recollection and Working Through. In *Collected Papers,* Vol. 2 Basic Books, New York, 1959.
16. Freud, S. Observations on Transference Love. In *Collected Papers,* Vol. 2, Basic Books, New York, 1959.

9

IRA MILLER

On Taking Notes

It is not unusual, during the course of free association, for a patient to enquire of the analyst, "Are you taking notes?" Certainly, in fanciful reproductions of the analytic situation such as cartoons, the analyst is identified by his notebook no less than by his beard and couch. When such a question is referred back to the analysand for his thoughts, almost invariably there is some association to the effect that the patient wants the analyst to take notes so as not to lose sight of a single, precious word.

That it is not advisable to take notes during an analytic hour is something with which most analysts would agree. This is based on the consideration that anything which distracts the analyst from the optimum free-floating attention interferes with the communciation, via the derivatives, between the unconscious of the analysand and the unconscious of the analyst (1). A perusal of the literature fails to reveal any mention of note-taking save in general terms. Glover (3), for example, states: ". . . note-taking is calculated either to arouse suspicion in the defensive type of patient or to give anxiety cases the impression, not altogether unfounded, that the analyst is unsure of himself." The purpose of this short communication is to delineate a specific resistance, both in the transference and countertransference, which may be served by the practice of taking notes. An attempt will be made to show that frequently the patient's professed "I don't want you to miss a single word" is penultimate to the unexpressed thought, "and at the same time not know what is

Reprinted from the *International Journal of Psychoanalysis*, 1964, Vol. 45, 121-122.

really going on," and that a similar resistance may be operative in the countertransference.

A middle-aged woman being seen in consultation following referral from another therapist, suddenly interrupted the anamnesis by stating, "You don't take notes. The other doctor wrote down everything I said—but perhaps you don't think it's that important. Anyway, I was more comfortable with him. You just sit there and look at me! I feel as though you're looking right through me and it makes me uneasy."

A 26-year-old graduate student asked, during the course of an hour, if the analyst were taking notes. When asked what thoughts he had about it, he first made some comments as to how the analyst couldn't remember so much if he didn't, and then added spontaneously, "When I'm in class listening to a lecture, I take notes furiously—but I don't know what really went on in the lecture until I can get home and read the notes over."

A university instructor once asked the same question, and when asked why he had asked, replied (after the usual associations about "How do you remember it all?", etc.) "This morning when I was lecturing I became very anxious. There was one student sitting at the back of the room who wasn't taking notes. The son-of-a-bitch just sat there and looked at me and I suddenly became very anxious when I had the thought, 'I wonder if he knows that I have homosexual thoughts?' "

It is clear from these illustrations that part of the feeling of comfort at the thought of the analyst's taking notes stems from a wish that the analyst shall not see what is going on *at the moment.* The instructor in the last illustration, for example, when this had been interpreted, stated that prior to asking the question about notes he had suddenly become very frightened that he might develop an erection while lying on the couch. It is not difficult to understand why he would have preferred such a feeling to be reduced to the level of an abstraction in the analyst's notebook.

The taking of notes, however, may have a meaning for the analyst as well. To illustrate this, I must tell of a personal experience in order to illustrate the operation of a counter-transference meaning to the process of taking notes. It is always difficult to write of such personal experiences, but if they can be of use to others, relating them is justified.

During the course of my analytic supervision work, it was my custom to write notes of the hours at some point later in the day. At one point in the treatment of a young woman, my supervisor indicated that things seemed to be going very well and suggested that the frequency of control sessions might be reduced. Following this consciously pleasurable bit of news, I suddenly found myself with a strong need to take notes on this particular patient during the analytic sessions. This procedure I rationalized on the basis of its saving time (despite the fact that I had just had some time set free) and that, since the supervision sessions were to be less frequent, I wanted to be certain not to forget anything important (again despite the fact that with fewer control sessions the need would be for less, rather than greater, detail). This note-taking continued, despite certain misgivings on my part, for about two weeks. At the next supervision session, the supervisor was able to point out several instances where I had overlooked manifestations of the transference, and stated, "I don't understand why you're missing this. You used not to." After leaving his office, I immediately connected this state of affairs somehow with the taking of notes, and, as I thought about it, the three incidents presented earlier in this paper came to mind. It suddenly became clear why this need had arisen within me and had allowed itself to be acted upon under the guise of such shallow rationalization. The announcement by the supervisor that the frequency of supervision hours could be reduced, had reawakened a facet of the oedipal conflict. The supervisor was stating, in effect, "She's all yours now," and my own anxiety was increased to the degree that I had to say, in effect, "No, she is not mine, father, she is still yours. I am only functioning as a go-between, carrying the transference directly to you via my notebook." As soon as this bit of countertransference became clear to me, the note-taking during the analytic hours stopped, and the analytic work was resumed from where it had been interrupted two weeks before.

This material is presented in order to show that the taking of notes *during* an analytic session will serve the resistance of the patient by virtue of its isolating and intellectualizing the associations, and that it may also be a manifestation of a defence on the part of the analyst by removing him from the impact of the transference.

It is sometimes easy to lose sight of the fact that the analytic situation is one which involves two people. Putting aside those situations where such an awareness is abused (as in some of the "wild" and undisciplined attempts to justify acting-out of the countertransference), it is important for the analyst to be able to allow his own unconscious a free, empathic rein. In a study of communication and the creative process, Beres (1) states,

> "The analyst is thus not a purely passive participant in this communicative relationship. In this he is indeed as the audience of the artistic creation. The analyst must be free to respond to the productions of the patient, to create in his own mind the images and feelings which correspond to those of the patient. . . .He collaborates in the creative process by supplying the skill of

> the poet to bring to the surface emotions and images (which are id derivatives) but to keep them controlled within the demands of the ego. . . . In the psychoanalytic interview specifically, communication between analysand and analyst plays a major role in breaking down the patient's resistances and preparing him for the insight and emotional experience that leads to conviction."

In this paper an attempt has been made to show that the taking of notes during the analytic process, *even though those notes concern the productions of the patient under consideration,* is a procedure which interferes with that communication between analyst and analysand so well described by Beres in the above quotation. That this is a procedure which may be welcomed by the resistances of both analyst and analysand has been illustrated. As most literary works suffer in translation, so the communication between analysand and analyst will suffer via the use of the analyst's notebook as an intermediary.

REFERENCES

1. Beres, David (1957). "Communication and the Creative Process." *J. Amer. Psychoanal. Assoc.*, 5.
2. Freud, S. (1912). "Recommendations to Physicians Practicing Psycho-Analysis." *S. E.*, 12.
3. Glover, Edward (1955). *The Technique of Psychoanalysis*. (New York: Int. Univ. Press.)

10

SANDOR S. FELDMAN

A Significant Comment Made by Patients When Relating their Dreams

"Everything is material" in analysis. One continuously discovers new proofs of it. Now and then some patients when relating a dream during a therapeutic session will say: "That's all" or "That's about all" or "That's all I can remember." They would say this in a somewhat apologetic way either before or after the dream is related. It is as if they were warning the analyst not to expect too much from the analysis of the dream, or as if they were trying to discourage the analyst. "After all, the dream was too short, why bother with it?" The patient seems to think that inasmuch as the dream is not all remembered and the dream is not complete, it does not have too much importance or cannot possibly be interpreted.

Of course this is all a resistance. But as Ernst Kris (1) justly reminds us, "Resistance is no longer simply an 'obstacle' to analysis, but part of the 'psychic surface' which has to be explored." Exploring such resistances is often a highly rewarding task. Through such explorations one learns how significant comments, such as those we mentioned, can be.

A man patient related the following dream: "I was going to make love to a girl but I couldn't do anything because my mother was around," and added, at the end, "That's all." Analysts hear similar dreams frequently. The manifest dream content might vary slightly here or there, but for our present task, this does not make any difference. The comment "That's all" is an immediate association to the dream and as such is quite valuable and as important as the latent dream thought. In this particular case, it means that this is all, that

Reprinted from *The Yearbook of Psychoanalysts*, 1953, Vol. 9, 109-112.

this is the core of his trouble, of his neurosis. Despite resistances, the dreamer reveals through such a comment the knowledge (negated or repressed in other ways) that the conflict hidden behind the dream is the clue to his neurosis. All other features of his illness are only complicating factors which appeared during the development of his neurosis. The relationship to his mother is where the trouble originated: that's all that counts.

> Another man patient, a practicing psychiatrist, told me one of his dreams. I had a dream, but it is vague. I dreamed that I awakened and realized that it was close to 10 o'clock and I had a patient at 10 o'clock in my office whom I have to hurry and see. But the patient, a man, is already here and my wife has let him come in. I am in my bathroom shaving and I assume an air of authority and while shaving I start the therapeutic session with him. Usually I use a Gillette Safety Razor, but this time I had a straight blade with an ivory handle. The screw which held the blade had gotten loose and I fixed it. In order to shave close I had to concentrate on the shaving and couldn't listen well to the patient, and if I concentrated on the patient, I couldn't have a good shave. I awakened. That's all I can remember.

The dreamer assumes (for reasons not necessary to be mentioned in this paper) the attitude that nothing is impossible for him to accomplish; he can cope with any situation. He thinks that a man who uses a straight razor blade is a "real he-man." Sometimes when he is bored by a patient, secretly he does something else and does not listen attentively. He even reads something. Once when he was doing this, the wish came into his mind that this should not come up during his analytic sessions: it would be embarrassing. The "loose screw" in the dream expresses self-criticism. He is guilty of loose conduct in his work. To silence the self-criticism, he is telling himself that he "can fix" everything. The "loose screw" of the dream refers furthermore to his fantasies of "screwing loosely," i.e., indiscriminately (which in reality he does not do).

The dreamer was right when he added to the dream, "That's all I can remember." In this case, it means (and this was proven in his analysis) that the dream content contains the core of his trouble, the neurotic part of his personality trouble; it means: "That's all it's necessary to remember." This colleague's social and professional attitude changed completely during his analysis.

A married woman patient related to me a dream which could be labeled a "That's about all dream." This patient suffers from attacks of paralyzing anxiety; she must always have near her a person who loves her. Because of her traumatic experiences in infancy and childhood she accepted, in her late girlhood, the advances of a motherly woman who admired, loved her and in many ways made up for the fact that her mother had frustrated her. But this new love relationship was far from satisfying. It made her feel abnormal, like a "monster." She felt extreme guilt about the whole thing and soon ceased seeing this woman. Shortly after the separation she developed severe attacks of anxiety. She feared that somehow or other her morbid relationship would be discovered, that her family would ostracize her. Even though she had completely stopped seeing the woman and her secret was not being uncovered, she felt unworthy and could not accept love from anybody, and without love her very existence was impossible and life intolerable to her.

The whole episode with this woman was not repressed but the connection between the anxiety and the episode had to be repressed, because through her anxiety, caused by this repression, she permitted herself to accept the kind support of a few people around her. The neurosis paralyzed her but without it she would have had to face a fact that she could not tolerate or live with.

> This was her state of mind when she had the following dream: I was in the town of X and I realized that my husband was not with me. He had gone out for a drive and left me alone. I was frightened and thought I would go to a relative (who had the same name as mine). When I arrived there I found many guests, dressed up, having a big party. I felt that she couldn't pay attention to me and therefore her presence wouldn't relieve my fright. I left to look for my husband and found him. Before this a woman accosted me on the street. She was investigating whether I am involved in subversive activities. I knew that I am innocent, that I am not a communist. She searched my handbag and there was a note with a cute content. She looked at me for an explanation, and I told her that this was a love note from my husband. We often exchange such cute love notes. That's about all.

Her great secret, the transitory sexual aberration, is represented in the dream as a secret subversive political activity which is persecuted by the government (like the sexual aberration is rejected by society). It is true that she is completely innocent in a political sense yet guilty in other ways. The patient got sick in the town of X. In reality the patient is very happily married and does exchange love notes with her husband. This and her normal sexual life in marriage (indicated in the dream by the handbag) works like an alibi against self-accusation for the past sexual abberation. Resistance distorts the sequence of events in the dream; it puts the fright at the beginning of the dream instead of at the end. The dream thought expresses one of her deepest concerns: "Because I was involved in secret sexual activities I am frightened, I feel guilty. I cannot be loved, accepted by my family and the community. That's about all—this is most of my trouble."

What makes patients express the truth without being aware of it? The truth has to come out because the secret, as Hermann explained, creates a gap between people and love cannot be enjoyed. The ego wants and needs love. But there is a great conflict. The secret prevents love, yet the removal of the secret is dangerous; should the secret be divulged love will be denied. The "That's about all" or "That's all" is a confession, but not a complete one–one part of the ego is unaware of what the other part is doing.

The author is interested in knowing whether other analysts can confirm or invalidate the correctness of this observation.

REFERENCES

1. Kris, Ernst: "Ego Psychology and Interpretation in Psychoanalytic Therapy." *Psychoanal. Quart., 20:* 18, 1951.

11

MARTIN H. ORENS

Setting a Termination Date: An Impetus to Analysis

In the course of any analysis the analytic situation itself begins at various times to take on very special meanings. On the conscious level patients come into therapy in order to be relieved of distressing symptoms and at the beginning of therapy this may be the main force that keeps them coming. However, somewhere in the course of analysis, particularly during those periods when they feel symptom free, there are probably other factors that keep them coming in the face of unpleasant reality of the time and money that is taken by the therapy itself. In spite of all our efforts to conduct the analysis in a spirit of abstinence, and in spite of all attempts to frustrate the transference wishes of the patient, there is a source of satisfaction that is difficult or impossible to stop and that is the unconscious satisfaction that probably every patient obtains from the analytic situation itself. This may be more or less apparent during the course of the analysis, but it is often very difficult for the patient to accept this as a satisfied wish, possibly because that understanding might mean the giving up of the satisfaction. There is one time, however, when this satisfaction is threatened without understanding or insight, and that is when the termination date for the analysis is agreed upon with the patient. These last weeks or months may be particularly fruitful because of the heretofore denied insight that can then be obtained.

I should like to present a patient in whom the analysis of this part of her psychic structure was not only very important to a more complete understanding of the patient but was vital for an under-

Reprinted with permission of the publisher from the *Journal of the American Psychoanalytic Association,* 1955, Vol. 3, 651-665.

standing of the main symptom. The patient is a twenty-four-year-old married woman who came into analysis with a complaint of severe depression which had been present for one year following the birth of her first child. When first seen, she seemed more sad than depressed. There were no suicidal fantasies, only slight loss of weight. She was neatly dressed and groomed. There was a general air of hopelessness about her with no retardation either psychically or physically.

She was the youngest of three siblings with two older brothers. At first she denied ever having had any symptoms before the onset of the depression, but it was soon evident that throughout her life she had had a number of mild, very transitory depressions because of her feelings of inferiority particularly in relation to her brothers. She was always in intense rivalry with them and always attempted to ape them, feeling very badly when she was unable to do so. Her main conscious goal was to obtain the favor of her father whom she felt could only love a complete person; that is a person who could do the things that her brothers could. She showed great ambivalence to her father. He was a rather successful man with a forceful personality, and for this he was greatly admired. She constantly sought his favor and remembered how often she would try to show off in front of him but she always had the feeling that he was paying little or no attention to her because of his favoring of the brothers who as boys could do more things than she could. The father was also a chronic alcoholic until recent years and he often came home almost unconscious at which time he would be completely taken care of by the mother. This was resented by the patient because she felt that it was at her expense.

The mother was described as a very warm loving person who was evidently somewhat of a martyr in regard to her father's drinking. She told the patient that it just had to be that way when the patient tried to induce the mother to be less concerned with the father when he was drunk. Her mother died when the patient was twenty years old, and soon she felt a pressing desire to get married and start a family. There were at this time conscious fantasies that now with her mother's death she would be the head female and she felt quite guilty about this. It became evident that one of the reasons for her desire to be married, was to break away from her father and deny the attachment to him that with her mother's death had become potentially dangerous of fulfillment.

She met a man a little older than herself and felt that she was in love. One year after her mother's death she married and became pregnant a year later of her own volition. Throughout the pregnancy she felt better than she had ever felt before in her life. She had none of the usual discomforts seen in most confinements and often had the conscious fantasy that it would be wonderful to be pregnant forever, because for the first time she felt equal to the rest of the world in all respects. She decided to have the delivery by natural childbirth for reasons that will be mentioned later. The delivery was accomplished without anesthesia and was a normal cephalic delivery. She was quite disappointed that the child was a girl because she was convinced that her father would only be pleased by grandsons and that he had no use for girls as daughters or grandchildren. She had noticed many conscious hostile thoughts to the child whom she blamed for the depression and stated a number of times that she had a recurring thought, "If you had not been born this would not have happened." Two days after the child's birth she began to feel depressed and remained this way until analysis started. She made no attempt to seek help before this because she had the conscious attitude that her illness was inevitable, and was just part and parcel of woman's lot in the world. Fortunately her younger brother was under analysis at the time and was doing quite well. He began to realize that his sister was sick and finally convinced her that it was not necessary for her to remain ill and that there was a possibility of help.

When she was first seen the predominant feeling was sadness and hopelessness. She repeated many times that the only possible solution was to become pregnant again because this was when she had felt so well. She more or less dismissed this as a temporary solution because after all she could not hope to remain pregnant forever. She was unconvinced that she could get well, and was sure that all women felt this way after childbirth, and therefore this reaction was just part of normal living. She was unconvinced that she was really ill and questioned whether analysis could ever help what she felt to be a normal reaction. The idea of entering therapy was the final admission of her worthlessness, and if people found out about it she would really be nothing in their eyes. It was mainly the realization that her brother had benefited from his analysis that finally induced her to start.

For about three months she refused to lie on the couch. She attempted this a number of times but within five minutes or so she would become panicky and have to sit up so that analysis was conducted for the most part in these months vis-a-vis. Although she never missed a session and was never late, she took the attitude that she was only coming to treatment because she had been told to and she made little or no attempt to even approximate free association. During this period most of the time was spent trying to understand the nature of her resistances to analysis and also to understand the panic states each time she approached the couch. For the most part the sessions of the first weeks took the form of questions and answers. The answers were very short and pointed and free of the usual associations that one would like to obtain from an analytic patient.

Particularly germane to the point of this paper was the gradually acquired knowledge that her fear of the couch was related in good part to the position itself, with the analyst above and behind her. She complained bitterly how helpless this made her feel and how powerless she was in this position. She had all kinds of fantasies as to the terrible sadistic acts that might be inflicted upon her by the analyst if she remained on the couch. She brought up a number of examples of people who had been hurt by psychoanalytic therapy and wondered whether analysts received any pleasure from that type of result. Conversely she feared her own hostility and was afraid to associate freely lest the release of her thoughts from conscious control damage the analyst. During the first weeks of analysis an interesting event occurred which is important in this regard. She mentioned very hesitatingly one day that her father-in-law was quite ill and that he might die in the near future. That afternoon when she came home from the session she found that he had died soon after the end of the session. For many sessions after that she was terrified to mention anything that could have a similar result. The next day in talking about the death she remarked that she felt as if her words had killed him. This was the first time in her analysis that she talked of "her bad influence on people." These sadomasochistic fantasies were worked through over and over again and eventually she was able to lie down and conduct analysis in the usual manner. Symptoms continued for ten months and then gradually disappeared. For the rest of the analysis she was symptom-free.

During analysis she became pregnant again. This time, although she felt quite well, she had more of the usual symptoms associated with normal pregnancy. She had another girl, but there was no depression, and she was not bothered by having had a second female child. We learned that she had attempted, but not successfully, to deny her absent penis. By identifying with her brothers and continually aping them she felt that she too had a penis. This was not a complete solution, for she did not really believe that she had a penis as was evidenced by her constant feelings of being inadequate and incomplete compared to the potent male. In addition she began to develop fantasies that she had gotten the penis from the male and had castrated him by this acquisition. The resultant punishment for this was to be horribly castrated in turn. Her picture of the relations between men and women was that of a horrible jungle with each one out to kill and maim the other. She was completely unprepared for her first menstrual period which started at the age of eleven during the night and she awoke to find her bedclothes blood-stained and consciously very unaware of what had happened to her. In her fantasies at the time, this was done in retaliation for her own castrative wishes by a male who had crept in during the night.

It is particularly interesting that many years later when she became pregnant she had the idea that she would like to have the baby via natural childbirth. She had a number of conscious reasons for this. She felt that it was more natural and better for the baby. She was particularly intrigued at the idea of no anesthesia because her mother had told her that it was a great thrill to be delivered without anesthesia and described it often to the patient as a very memorable experience. The patient stated, "So I did what my mother had done; I admired her a good deal and one of my main impulses was to live up to her and be like her." Actually unconsciously she was terrified at the idea of being put to sleep again, as she had been at the age of eleven, and again castrated by a male, the obstetrician. This was also a factor in her early inability to lie on the couch at the beginning of the analysis. It was very important that she remain awake and alert and so prevent any recurrence of the previously experienced sadistic attacks upon her. Gradually it became clear that in spite of her precautions to avoid recastration, the actual delivery was experienced as the loss of the penis with the usual equating of child and phallus. She had many fantasies in the beginning of the analysis that perhaps her delivery had not been as normal as she had been told. She thought that her doctor had made some serious mistake which she was not told about, and the resultant physical damage was the real cause of the depression. This was also related to the analyst who might also make a mistake and cause her to be even sicker than she was.

It seemed that one of the main factors in the causation of the depression was this loss of the fantasied penis; but then the question arose as to why it had not happened after the second delivery. She had a few more of the usual physical complaints with the second pregnancy as compared to the first, but again she felt quite well. The delivery was again by natural childbirth and again there was a normal cephalic delivery with no anesthesia. She said many times just before and just after the delivery that she was not convinced that she was really cured, but it might be the fact that she was still under analysis that had prevented another depression. She talked often of her more or less conscious desire to be perpetually pregnant. She expressed the thought that this was one way in which she could beat men at their own game. The baby was not only her substitute for a penis, but it was an even bigger penis than the man could ever hope to have.

There was little doubt that this second pregnancy was in part at least an acting out under pressure of the transference in relation to her wishes to be impregnated by the analyst who in turn was her father. This became very clear when in the early part of the pregnancy she became very concerned about the analyst's health and often expressed her feeling that as she blossomed out in pregnancy the analyst was waning and she felt very guilty about this. There was always a balance of potency between the patient and the male object of the moment. It was noteworthy that during the period that she was feeling quite well, particularly after the second pregnancy, she became very concerned about the state of her husband's emotional health and she repeatedly urged him to be analyzed. She noted many times how strange it was that she got well at the same time that her husband seemed to become ill. She compared herself to the female spider who eats the male after impregnation because then the male is castrated and worthless. During pregnancy she had many dreams which could be easily interpreted as dreams of perpetual pregnancy. She compared her feeling after the first delivery to the way Christine Jorgenson must have felt after the operation. She felt that she did not have this after the second delivery because of the analysis. She stated that each session was like an injection by a physician and that these injections were necessary to keep her going. She had many prostitution fantasies as another way of getting the penis; however, there were strong defenses against these fantasies. She had gotten married partly with the conscious idea that this would be the best safeguard against promiscuity, and she vehemently condemned unfaithfulness in anyone.

She continued to feel well after the second delivery, and after a number of months she began to talk of ending the analysis. Associated with this was a moderate slowing in the flow of material with occasional silences intervening. She decided to test herself during the summer vacation. When she returned she reported that her symptoms had not returned and even her old feelings of inferiority had vanished and she requested discharge from therapy. The analyst agreed to termination but requested that she remain for three more months. Her first response was to be happy about the end of the analysis, but then she requested that the three-month period be waived because she felt so well and she was sure that nothing further could be gained. This was analyzed as a resistance and about two weeks later it became clear that she did not really wish to leave therapy and that she still felt that analysis was essential to her well-being. She began to be troubled with the idea that since discharge meant that she was healthy, it also meant correspondingly the death of the analyst. She fantasied that with the end of her analysis the analyst would have to give up his practice and no longer function as an analyst. It was very difficult to induce her to associate to this, but in general she felt that she had been a difficult patient and that she had taken so much out of the analyst by getting well that naturally he would have nothing left for anyone else. Then she had a dream: "I am pregnant again and am about ready to deliver the baby; I was in the delivery room but I was not in labor; I was told that my obstetrician was temporarily unavailable; I don't know why, but there was a feeling that he had left practice because of illness. I said that I would only allow him to deliver me and they told me that it might mean that I would never be delivered and I said, 'so what' but felt a little nervous." In associating she was sure that this had something to do with the termination of therapy and that the analysis itself was like being pregnant because the regular visits to the analyst were like the regular visits to the obstetrician and so the analyst was the absent obstetrician of the dream. If the obstetrician could not deliver her it meant that the pregnancy would go on forever and thus the analysis would never terminate. The end of analysis was like a delivery and meant that she would again be castrated and worthless. The illness of the obstetrician reminded her of her concern about the health of the analyst during the second pregnancy and as long as he remained ill he could not perform the delivery, that is the castration. At this time she talked a good deal about the actual time of delivery. The moment that she feared most was just before the delivery when the baby was about to come out. She had often wondered what prevented sudden explosive delivery of the baby with resultant physical damage to the mother. She had a conscious fear of bursting from the pressure of the undelivered baby. This brought her to the subject of explosive diarrhea after being constipated. She had been toilet trained at the age of two with little difficulty. She did not bring up any material to show that this was particularly traumatic. She has had infrequent episodes of constipation and has had momentary concerns that if the stool got too big she would be damaged when she eventually did have a movement. It is also important to note that when she was two, her father fell and sustained a severely fractured leg from which he never recovered completely and he limps to this day. She has always felt somewhat guilty about this injury, although realistically she has never been able to implicate herself in any way.

She felt quite proud of the mastery of her bowels. This material was not obtained from recollections of the patient concerning herself but was seen in her attitude to her older child who was being bowel trained during the analysis. The child was two years old. Her identification with the daughter during this period was clear and she often remarked how proud the girl must feel to be able to acquire this control. She then said rather wistfully, "I guess she is no longer a baby now but is a big girl." Evidently this control over the bowels was a form of potency which later became connected in her mind with the injury to her father which happened at the same time that she achieved this potency. She got the idea that she could only achieve potency at the expense of the male being castrated.

At this time in reporting a dream she began the session by emphasizing her husband's need for analysis. She felt that, like her father, he was starting to drink too much. The night of the dream she had strongly urged him to start therapy as soon as possible "for his own sake." She then reported: "I was having intercourse with my husband and right after it I began to bleed profusely. There was blood all over the floor and I was mopping it up with a sponge." Her first thoughts were again about the fact that now with the end of the analysis approaching she was feeling so well and her husband seemed to be sicker than ever. In talking of the dream she said, "In the dream my husband makes me sick which is the opposite of what I have been talking about. He makes me into a bleeding woman. The sponge reminds me of times when I used to wipe up the feces of a pet dog who was not yet toilet trained." She was able to compare bleeding from the vagina with an uncontrolled bowel movement. The equation of lack of bowel control with menstruation and castration became clearer. To bleed is the complete confirmation of castration, as is the loss of bowel control.

During these last months there were two major changes in the character of the analysis. Before the termination date was set most of the material was on phallic levels. This centered about the castration complex with the loss of the phallus in the form of the baby at the time of delivery as the seeming main cause for the depression plus the fact that the child was a girl which made it a worthless gift for her father. During this time the transference for the most part was such that the analyst represented her father to her. After the termination date was set there was a good deal of preoedipal material which had not been mentioned before and the transference seemed to be mostly related to her mother.

The reconstruction of the events in this case would appear to be as follows. It is evident that her first menstrual period was rather traumatic. She regressed to anal levels and interpreted the flow of blood as uncontrolled fecal discharge. Coincident with this regression was a welling up of sadistic impulses and fantasies normally associated with the anal period of development. She considered her bowel training to be a form of potency which with the onset of menstruation was lost. She began to blame herself for the injury to her father, and it was as if from that time her potency could only be obtained at the expense of the male. From then on she did all that she could to protect the male from her sadism. She compared herself not only to the female spider but also said that she must have the kiss of death in her because in the past few years she had had three male pets killed in accidents. In reference to her husband and father she said, "I am so afraid to hurt them that I never say anything against them even when I am right." She attempted to prevent too close contact with the male at all times for his protection. This was clearly seen in the transference, in the beginning of the analysis, when she was very careful to keep the analyst in his place as the therapist with whom she really had no close contact. This was also seen in her manner of dress. She was neatly dressed at all times, but there was obviously no attempt made to enhance her natural feminine attractiveness. During the course of analysis this changed and she began to appear in very feminine outfits. About this she said, "I might have hurt men by being too inviting and attractive; I used to be afraid they would think wrong things about me if I dressed this way." Deutsch (2) has written rather extensively on the relation between the first menstrual period and the female castration complex. She also emphasizes the increase of aggressivity during the menstrual period.

The patient then desired the phallus and defended strongly against these wishes. She became pregnant partly in an attempt to satisfy this wish. She felt exceptionally well during the pregnancy because she had the longed-for phallus, but then delivery was interpreted as a castration and most probably was felt like the first menstrual period. She regressed to earlier levels and again reactivated her aggressiveness. It would be far beyond the scope of this paper to delve into the psychopathology of the depressive symptom itself, which has been discussed by so many different authors from so many different viewpoints. Bibring (1) has stressed the importance of the loss of self-esteem for whatever reason it may have occurred. This certainly played an important role in this patient. With the delivery she became not only the worthless castrated creature, but the gift she had readied for her father was also worthless. Again it may be worth noting as was mentioned before, that the presenting symptom as related by the patient was depression, but clinically she appeared to have more of a feeling of hopelessness than depression.

Then because of the depression she came into analysis. Her symptoms gradually disappeared and she became pregnant again and delivered another girl, but this time there was no depression even with a repeat of the castration. It became evident that there was something about the analysis itself that acted as a nullification of the castration induced by the delivery.

At this point one wonders about the origin of the penis envy in this woman. Deutsch (2) has emphasized that "Penis envy is not a primary factor but a secondary one." Jones (3) feels that the sight of the boy's penis is only the last link in a long chain. This patient spent her adult life in pursuit of the elusive phallus, but to get it always meant destruction of the male. About one year after the start of the analysis she had the following dream: "Everyone has been poisoned; my father, husband, child, brothers; only my mother and myself are left alive." She associated as follows: "I am not sure who did the poisoning, but I have the uncomfortable feeling that I was responsible. As a result I am left alone with my mother and I guess in many ways that is what I want. It would be a completely parasitic condition where I would be completely taken care of. I guess that is when life is best; there are no worries. I suppose the only time that that is true is before we are born. I killed everyone off in the dream because they were all rivals for my mother; the worst rival was father because he was drunk so often and had to be taken care of like a little child. I guess I was really complete only when I was still attached to my mother." The idea of being complete only when she was attached to her mother brings to mind the often expressed complaint during analysis that she was incomplete because she did not have a penis. One wonders whether or not the idea that lack of a penis was incompleteness was not a later construction derived from the incompleteness that she felt as the result of her separation from her mother after the oral period. All her rivals for mother were realistically males and perhaps it is from this that she got the idea that the penis was so necessary for this reunion with her mother.

When she became pregnant on one level she attained the desired phallus and so she felt fine and complete. In addition we have seen how much she identified with her mother during this pregnancy. Deutsch (2) has emphasized that the expectant mother identifies both with her own mother and the future child and the "fear of separation is not only that I am losing the child but the child is losing me." So it may be that the original phallus was in fantasy the attachment to her mother which later was displaced to the possession of the penis. Psychologically this was a double pregnancy, her own and her mother's. Delivery was then not only a castration like the first menstrual period but was also experienced as a repeat of her own birth; the original separation from mother.

The place of the analysis in all this was not found out until this patient had been given a definite termination date. Then it was seen that in spite of what she consciously felt she did not wish to leave analysis. Analysis was the longed-for perpetual pregnancy in which she was able to get not only the penis but was also able to be reunited with her mother. Thus the end of the analysis is not only her castrating delivery again but is also her own birth and the dreaded separation from mother.

Eventually the symptomatology could be understood on at least two levels. On the phallic level it was mainly related to the female castration complex. For the major part of the analysis this was the main theme. The symptoms disappeared with the analysis of this material. However, it was only when she was given a termination date which acted like a frustration of the transference that the symptomatology could be understood on preoedipal levels as well and was seen to be very importantly related to her attachment to her mother.

Discussion

This patient was presented as an example of the importance of ascertaining in as much detail as possible the actual unconscious meaning of the analysis to the patient as well as the meaning of the end of the analysis. Although each patient, consciously at least, wants to get well and earnestly seeks the end of a successful analysis, it must always be remembered that this conscious wish may be outweighed by the unconscious satisfactions that the analysis itself may give and that this may result in a serious resistance to the end of analysis. Nunberg (4) has stated: "We can never calculate the probable duration and success of analytic treatment from the conscious wish to get well. Every psychoanalyst knows that those neurotics who are so impatient that they can hardly wait for the beginning of treatment are not the easiest ones to treat." He emphasizes the fact that the word "cure" means different things to the analyst and the unconscious of the patient, and states:

> There is invariably a misunderstanding in those who undergo analysis; . . . the analysand expects from psychoanalysis something other than it can give." He feels that the desire for recovery always originates in the instinctual life of early infancy and says, "Thus the wish to get well, which is nourished from the unconscious, makes use of the transference in order to attain in the present the infantile instinctual aims. . . . The desire to get well impels the patient to undergo treatment; the transference is merely the means used . . . . The wish to get well is essentially the antithesis of cure in the sense of an adaptation to reality, for the aim of the desire is to restore an infantile libido-position. . . . Yet this desire is indispensable for the success of the treatment." He makes a point of the fact that "The desire to get well does not arise if in the symptoms the actual unpleasure is either wholly balanced by the attainment of a corresponding degree of primary pleasure, as for

instance in cases of masochism. . . . In all these cases treatment, if it does not actually fail, is made very much more difficult. Thus a patient cannot be treated at all against his own will.

This patient started analysis more or less against her own will, and yet she made definite progress. I think that this can be explained by assuming her reluctance to be analyzed as a defense wherein she could not be held responsible for the result of the analysis because after all as she said she was only coming because she was told to do so. The stimulus given to this patient by suggesting termination of the analysis elicited a wealth of material helping to bring out findings on deeper levels than had heretofore been the case. The frustration of transference wishes is one of the most important tools in any analysis to help push the analysis to deeper and deeper levels. In this patient a most important transference frustration was obtained when she knew that her analysis was about to end.

Summary

A patient was presented who came into analysis with a postpartum depression of one year's duration. In the course of the analysis it was found that her most pressing problems had to do with the female castration complex. During analysis she had a second child with no depression. She requested discharge and was given a definite termination date. The threat of separation from the analysis caused a flow of previously unknown material, and deeper levels of the unconscious were uncovered. The importance of finding out the meaning of the analytic situation and the end of the analysis was stressed.

REFERENCES

1. Bibring, E. The Mechanism of Depression. In: *Affective Disorders*, ed. P. Greenacre. New York: International Universities Press, 1953.
2. Deutsch, H. *The Psychology of Women*, 2 Vols. New York: Grune & Stratton, 1944, 1945.
3. Jones, E. The Early Development of Female Sexuality. *Papers on Psychoanalysis.* Baltimore: William & Wilkins, 1948.
4. Nunberg, H. The Will to Recovery. In: *Practice and Theory of Psychoanalysis*. New York: International Universities Press, 1955.

12

SANDOR LORAND with
WILLIAM A. CONSOLE

Therapeutic Results in Psychoanalytic Treatment Without Fee

In an address given before the Fifth International Psychoanalytic Congress at Budapest in September, 1918, Freud made the following inspiring remarks:

> And now in conclusion I will cast a glance at a situation which belongs to the future—one that will seem fantastic to many of you, but which I think, nevertheless, deserves that we should be prepared for it in our minds. You know that the therapeutic effects we can achieve are very inconsiderable in number. We are but a handful of people, and even by working hard each one of us can deal in a year with only a small number of persons. Against the vast amount of neurotic misery which is in the world, and perhaps need not be, the quantity we can do away with is almost negligible. Besides this, the necessities of our own existence limit our work to the well-to-do classes, accustomed to choose their own physicians, whose choice is diverted away from psychoanalysis by all kinds of prejudices. At present we can do nothing in the crowded ranks of the people who suffer exceedingly from neuroses.
>
> Now let us assume that by some kind of organization we were able to increase our numbers to an extent sufficient for treating large masses of people. Then, on the other hand, one may reasonably expect that at some time or other the conscience of the community will awake and admonish it that the poor man has just as much right to help for his mind as he now has to the surgeon's means of saving life: and that the neuroses menace the health of a people no less than tuberculosis, and can be left as little as the latter to the feeble handling of individuals. Then clinics and consultation departments will be built, to which analytically trained physicians will be appointed, so that the men who would otherwise give way to drink, the women who have nearly succumbed under their burden of privations, the children for whom there is no chioce but running wild or neurosis, may be made by analysis able to resist

Reprinted from the *International Journal of Psychoanalysis,* 1958, Vol. 39, 59-64.

and able to do something in the world. This treatment will be free. It may be a long time before the State regards this as an urgent duty. Present conditions may delay its arrival even longer; probably these institutions will first be started by private beneficence; some time or other, however, it must come.

One direct result of these words was the opening of the Berlin Psychoanalytic Clinic in February 1920. In his report on the operation of this clinic, Eitingon indicated that while many patients paid the maximum that they could afford, there were some who were completely without means and were treated free of any charge. No mention is made of the length of time of the gratuitous therapy.

In May 1922 the Viennese Psychoanalytic Ambulatorium was opened. Here, according to Hitschman's report, each member of the Viennese Psychoanalytic Society took one or more patients at the start. While it is not specified, this is interpreted to mean that the doctor received no payment for his work but each patient paid a small fee. At the Berlin Clinic many of the patients were treated in the Psychoanalytic Clinic Building and a number of them in the doctors' private offices. In Vienna the larger part of the patients received their treatment in the doctors' own offices.

The London Clinic of Psychoanalysis was opened on Freud's seventieth birthday, 1926. Then other clinics were opened at Budapest and on the European continent.

The problem of the patient paying for his therapy, the importance of payment, and the arrangement of the payments has been dealt with by many observers in the psychoanalytic literature. However, patients who did not pay any fee for their treatment and the problems involved in not paying, as also the results with patients who did not pay any fee, are mentioned only by Freud himself.

The difficulties thought by many to be inherent in psychoanalysis without fee are as follows:

The patient does not "bring a sacrifice," which leads to barriers, since the money has multiple unconscious and symbolic meanings for him as well as its being a reality factor.

Not paying seriously interferes with the patient's ability to deal with his conflicts about *getting, possessing*, and *giving*.

The transference neurosis could not be handled adequately because the patient would shy away from displaying negative feelings so as not to anger the analyst.

The patient would become unnecessarily dependent on the analyst, and would be rendered unable to acquire the self-reliance and independence in the transference, which represents the ultimate goal of the therapy.

In addition to these supposed difficulties which militate against psychoanalysis without fee, further complicating factors have to be considered. There are still the problems attendant upon the therapist's not being paid and those arising from payment being made by someone other than the patient.

These objections, though valid to a certain degree, cannot be sustained as a whole. In elaboration of this problem, Freud (in his paper, "Further Recommendations in the Technique of Psychoanalysis on Beginning the Treatment," 1913, from *Collected Papers*, Volume 2) writes:

> Then the question arises whether the advantage to the patient (of gratuitous treatment) would not outweigh the physician's sacrifice. I may rely on my own judgement in this matter, since I have given an hour daily, and sometimes two, for ten years to gratuitous treatment, because I wished, for the purpose of studying the neuroses, to work with the fewest possible hindrances. The advantages which I sought in this way were not forthcoming. Gratuitous treatment enormously increases the transference relationship for young women, or the opposition to the obligatory gratitude in young men arising from the father-complex, which is one of the most troublesome obstacles to the treatment. The absence of the corrective influence in payment of the professional fee is felt as a serious handicap; the whole relationship recedes into an unreal world; and the patient is deprived of a useful incentive to exert himself to bring the cure to an end.
>
> In the same essay he cautions: Naturally, one does occasionally meet with people who are helpless from no fault of their own, in whom unpaid treatment leads to excellent results without exciting any of the difficulties mentioned.

The first extensive experience with free psychoanalytic treatment was begun in America in 1950 with the establishment of the Psychoanalytic Clinic of the State University Medical Center. With the help of the Professor and Chairman of the Department of Psychiatry this clinic was set up to be operated by the Psychoanalytic Faculty of the University as an integral part of the psychoanalytic training of the residents and staff members of the Psychiatric Division. For technicolegal reasons no fee could be charged, so that the treatment of all patients accepted for psychoanalysis was given without charge. The candidates in training who treated these patients and saw each of them four or five times weekly for fifty-minute sessions were in part compensated for their work by receiving their weekly and biweekly supervisory sessions individually without cost to them.

The supervising analysts were paid by the University for their supervision of those cases treated without charge in the clinic. In this way both the doctor who treated the patient and the doctor who supervised the patient's treatment were compensated for their time and work to a more or less fair degree. The lecturers and seminar leaders were paid by the University for each hour they spent in instruction.

The free treatment continued for about two or three years by the same therapist in the clinic. The candidate in training has usually finished his required four-year curriculum in the Psychoanalytic Institute by that time and he is exempt from further work in the clinic setting. He then arranges for transferring his clinic patients (who are usually two in number) to his private office for further treatment if the patient is in an economic position to pay a small fee and is willing or has the need to continue analysis. This arrangement, to our observation so far, works out very satisfactorily. It is discussed with the patients in the clinic many months ahead, and arrangements about fees which are acceptable to the patient's material circumstances are made.

There are many problems which may ensue with patients treated without charge in such a clinical setting which may not be present in office treatment; they do not create more hardship in the way of therapy, but the problems present themselves in a different way. For instance, the patients know each other, they meet constantly in a common waiting room, the patients know that their therapists are at the same time candidates in the Psychoanalytic Institute, and they know that their therapy is supervised by a senior member of the Psychoanalytic Faculty. But this atmosphere became a favorable one to the psychoanalytic therapy and, just as in any private office, the positive and negative transference reactions became the center and the topic of the analytical therapy in the private treatment rooms of the Psychoanalytic Clinic. It is true that some transference problems in the course of the therapeutic process came up, which may have been expressed differently than they would have been had the patient been treated in the doctor's private office. In the atmosphere of the clinic, since the patient was not paying for the treatment, his expression of certain feelings may have been delayed for a while. As one of the patients expressed it, since she was not paying she would have to be very careful about how she reacted to the doctor's feelings She has to be careful in any demonstration of any feelings because she would be rebuffed and dismissed from the treatment. She said, "Only if you pay for treatment can you have the privilege of making demands upon your doctor." On occasion the same patient attacked the analyst, telling him that if she were a paying patient she would not be refused medicine and made to suffer.

But even with paying patients we have the experience that some of them do delay talking about many matters, about resentments especially, and some about sexual matters relating to the analyst. The analyst has to be alert enough to pick up references to these problems directly or to understand the symbolic references to such material in dreams. The clinic patients did dream about money and bring up economic problems quite early in the analysis, but the analyst often missed it and did not report it in his supervisory session either, and so the material was lost and time had to elapse until the patient brought up the same material again. Then the analyst, being more alert and aware of it, handled adequately the material produced.

With certain patients we could ascribe to their not paying for treatment, as mentioned above, certain anxieties, hesitancies about bringing forth material pertaining to the transference relationship directly as freely and as early as patients who are treated in private offices and are paying for their analysis. Some patients, for instance, felt that being selected from a number of applicants for free clinic treatment meant that they were "privileged" and selected as research cases and that they had to be on their best behavior. If their doubts about the analyst's competence came up (which they connected with the idea that if he were not paid he could not be good) they didn't dare mention it for a time but did mention it in a later phase of analysis, usually in the second year when they are better able to express their criticism, aggression, and dissatisfaction. They could also bring up the problem that they really have no right to complain because they are not paying anything. However, this thought, as they admitted, was there for a long stretch of time before they were able to bring it up. One patient, in her aggressive mood, complained of her insecurity in not having a permanent analytical room assigned to her and because at times she had to change to another room. After a long period of silence, when it was brought to her attention that she was probably resisting because of annoyance at this shifting of rooms and that she might try to talk more about the matter, she said, "I feel I must talk. I am not entitled *not to talk* because I don't pay you and if I won't talk you will hate me because you probably hate me anyhow for not paying."

Another patient, in a mood of dissatisfaction with the progress of her analysis, expressed her lack of progress as follows; "I am paying nothing so I will get nothing." This patient also later expressed her resentment that she had to come to a free clinic at the very outset. She had no say about the choice of the doctor, or the choice of the time, as do patients who pay. Naturally, this problem brought up the whole complex material about being underprivileged, etc. This type and similar material were listed in the course of therapy, which led to working through more effectively the negative feelings in the transference parallel with the always present basic positive attitude and relationship.

One patient, who for months was full of gratitude for having free analysis, slowly began to talk about the embarrassment of coming to a charity clinic. When it was explained to him (which he knew anyhow) that he is really not a charity case because he pays taxes and the clinic of the University is maintained by the State and his taxes contribute to maintenance costs, he continued with his annoyance and irritation because he has to accept "being one of the poor people and also has to accept treatment by clinic doctors who are never really interested in the patients." In the further progress of his analysis, this patient interestingly expressed the early feelings which he never talked about until the second year of his analysis to the effect that when he originally came to the clinic he had felt that he was putting something over on the analyst by concealing his savings and had felt in constant danger of being found out and dismissed. Interestingly enough also, his analyst should have had an inkling about it, because the first dream he reported early in his analysis was, "I put a nickel in a vending machine and a handful of money came out of it." Furthermore, he continued talking in this aggressive vein, commenting that the clinic is a "cut-rate joint" and also that his treatment "accomplishes nothing." On the other hand, parallel to this type of thoughts there was always the fear of being expelled from the clinic by the "arbitrary, cruel and deceitful doctor." This patient also rationalized in another manner (which was partly true). He is really paying for his treatment. Why? First, by paying withholding taxes from which the State and the Federal governments benefit. Secondly, he cannot work overtime and is deprived of additional earnings because he has to come to the clinic. Thirdly, by using his car he is wearing out the tires and the engine which become depreciated, all because he has to drive to the clinic. This type of reaction and, in general, direct criticism of the analyst and censuring association and thoughts in the early phases of analysis, were quite a common occurrence. Some of the patients looked upon the common waiting room as an embarrassing place, many being afraid of what the other people would think of them and feeling humiliated. Others had the feeling at times that they were spied on by the other patients. They expressed the hatred of having to sit on those benches and felt hurt, which they then expressed directly against the analyst since he was the one who made them feel unimportant and low. One of the patients, in discussing this situation, exclaimed, "I wish I were paying you. I would just stop paying and would punish you that way and walk out." I must say that this type of reaction was not different, on the whole, from the reactions which we find in cases in private practice.

The patient's not paying caused some difficulties to the analyst, and the supervisory analyst had to be constantly alert to the necessity for maintaining the interest of the analyst in this problem of his patient, which quite often did escape the therapist's attention. First, because the analyst, though being partially compensated for treating his patient in the clinic (this was mentioned above), still had to bring sacrifices, and realistically had certain hardships in continuing to treat his patient in the clinic and coming to the clinic for that special reason. This was true of all our candidates in training to a milder degree, and some of them consciously felt it very costly and unconsciously, as was natural, more so.

There was also the problem of the open interest in a certain type of case and the material produced by those cases and their lack of interest in other types of material and in the cases themselves. Conscious of this, we tried to select the first and second patient for each and every candidate according to what we knew about the analyst's ability and his suitability to treat certain cases. Some of the young therapists were easily prone to interpret certain aspects of the patients' productions, certain dreams, and neglected other types of material, and some picked out deep symbolic material for interpretation and pushed aside obvious reality problems and transference material, among them the question of paying or not paying.

The handling of the negative transference of the patient sometimes elicited serious counter-transference manifestations in the analyst. In such situations some of them were likely to show a rigidity to the patient, following the mirror-like attitude too strictly. The aim was to control the patient and his attitude, also to control themselves from displaying any feelings of antagonism to the patient's aggression, and such an attitude came from unrecognized counter-transference feelings. A common example, for instance, was when the therapist did not interpret the patient's aggressivity which was brought to his attention many times by the patient's constant repetition of his plans for a weekend, or plans which may have involved a great deal of "acting out." The reason for not interpreting was admittedly anxiety on the analyst's part that the patient might do something desperate if all the unconscious involvements in his plans were interpreted to him. In the analyst's mind, the patient was not ready for the interpretation. Such attitudes showed themselves more frequently in candidates who had characterological problems referring to strong narcissistic feelings, feelings of power which enhance the gratification of the analyst in relationship to the patient's dependence. This certainly resulted in withdrawal from seeing the transference situation clearly. It was easy to trace back such a defensive attitude to the therapist's unconscious feelings of guilt in relationship to the feelings about his patient. Usually such difficulties in the analyst were eliminated in his own analysis, which was still in process at the time of the occurrence of such behavior. Such counter-transference feelings of the analyst usually did not much disturb the analytical or therapeutical process, because the analyst was under supervision, and it could be taken care of before acting and behaving in a manner which would endanger the continuation of analysis and the progress of cure became a permanent pattern in the analyst. The supervisory analyst handled such manifestation of counter-transference actings and behavior as he had to; namely as transitory because they were amenable to correction in the candidate's own analysis.

For some, the therapy and working with the patient represented too much satisfaction. This was the type of thing that happened with analysts whom we find being over-zealous, very ambitious to cure their patients, and very impatient with the progress of therapy if the patient did not progress rapidly enough. They very often missed practical problems and concentrated on transference relationship for their own unconscious gratification, playing rôles and manipulating the patient. They could not be sufficiently objective. Behind this over-ambitiousness was a great deal of anxiousness and insecurity which often led to acting out in relationship to the patient.

In general, this problem was the same as is found with all the candidates who begin therapy in supervision. Some interpreted the patient's feelings about the analyst and analysis in early sessions. Others postponed interpretation of transference. Some interpreted the transference when the original emotional situations were relived and re-experienced in relationship to the analyst. It was for the constant alertness of the supervisory analyst (as it has to be with those first cases in supervision) to direct the candidate's attention to such problems.

The analyst's drive to be important and independent, which he feels the need to express in the therapeutic situation (and this was a common experience in our candidates), proved always to be a characterological defence due to counter-transference.

The counter-transference manifestations were at times maintained by the fact of the candidate's being still involved in his own analysis during the time that he was treating his own patients analytically, and the candidate was therefore more prone to project his own problems in the relationship with his patients.

It was natural for the candidates who had already finished their four-year curriculum requirements to be annoyed about making four trips per week to the Psychoanalytic Clinic, which was located at the University, solely for the purpose of treating the free patients. They were all eagerly looking forward to the time when they could transfer their patients to their private offices. The candidates' feelings about money, the patient's not paying, and their not being sufficiently compensated at times entered into their relationship with the patient. The supervisor found good opportunities to point out such problems, which were real to some extent. The candidate doing the analysis became more aware of his counter-transference problems on a conscious basis. The realistic awareness helped to prevent him from "acting out." However, if they created deeper problems, they could be referred to the candidate's own analyst. This then led to a deeper insight and the candidate slowly reached a higher degree of stability and emotional health. He gained a deeper insight which made him more able to analyze his patients more effectively. It increased his alertness and self-scrutiny, and he slowly learned to become an impartial mediator between the patient's conscious and unconscious.

The supervisory analysts had varied feelings about the problem of free treatment. Fifteen senior analysts worked in a supervisory capacity with twenty-eight candidates, each of whom were treating one or two patients at the same time. The attitude of almost all the supervisors regarding the free treatment was that it can be carried out in the same way as in supervision of candidates who work with patients in their offices. However, they felt that it calls for more alertness at times and that certain candidates who themselves had not progressed far enough in their own analyses to have a more healthy type of counter-feelings in relation to their patients, sometimes had disturbing counter-transference manifestations. One supervisor had felt strongly that not charging a fee is definitely contra-indicated because it creates complications in the treatment which should be avoided. Such a feeling on the part of the supervisory analyst naturally caused the candidate (who had a latent feeling of the same type) to display a strong counter-feeling in the analytical situation, at times a negative attitude about the patient and about the treatment. Another time, the supervisor felt that even though gratuitous treatment may be undertaken, just as soon as the patient can afford to pay he should be transferred to the candidate's private office even if the payment there should only amount to a token fee. This supervisor's overall attitude was that the treatment would be facilitated if the patients were to pay "some sort of a fee." Some supervisors felt that if the patients had paid in the clinic for their therapy, the analysis would have proceeded at a much faster pace. The thought behind such feelings was that if the patient had been in a position to "make more sacrifices," he would have felt the frustrations more keenly, would have felt less dependent on the analyst and less protected in the analytical situation.

In spite of all the difficulties above mentioned, we must state that the difficulties encountered in this new milieu of treating the patients without charge were very little different from the general difficulties which are found in the office practice. The reports of the supervisory analysts about the treatment which they conducted showed that the difficulties were only somewhat different quantitatively and not qualitatively. The patients' emotional conflicts became externalized, explored and made amenable for resolving their difficulties to a considerable degree.

In the process of analysis, it was found that most of the patients whom we accepted for free analysis could have paid a low or a token fee in the Psychoanalytic Clinic from the inception of their therapy. However, as I mentioned above, for technical reasons we could not charge any fee. As it turned out, all of them so far made considerable progress in the course of their treatment in the clinic, some of them even with striking results in the sphere of their environmental, social, and work life, and partly in their sexual adjustment. In those two or three years of free analysis, the level on which the patients showed most progress was in the better behavior in their social life and in their work. Patients whose desire to work was negligible developed more need to support themselves, to be independent and earn more. The majority of them made considerable progress in securing better jobs and having some savings, so that when their transfer to private treatment was discussed, while there was some rebellion against it, to a large extent there was very little difficulty in accepting continuance of their treatment on a paying basis. For example, to mention one of our patients, a girl who was sent from one of the psychiatric centers where she obtained some psychotherapy, who was referred to our clinic because she could not afford any fee for analysis and was in need of it. She has now had three years of free analysis, and not only has she secured a permanent job, but she has turned out to be a very capable and reliable person, so that she is at present earning five thousand dollars a year. Her analyst will soon finish his fourth year in the Psychoanalytic Institute and will transfer her, as a paying patient, to his private office.

A patient, after transfer to private office treatment, may pay as little as \$25 or \$50 on a monthly basis for four or five weekly analytical sessions. Up to the present, our experience is that the greater part of the patient's time spent in treatment is in the clinic setting, free of charge, and another part, which is usually of shorter duration, on the low-fee basis in the analyst's office.

The overall nature of our clinical material was as follows: From January 1, 1951, to March 31, 1956, fifty-nine patients received free treatment in the Psychoanalytic Clinic of the State University. Diagnostically they represented what one would expect following careful screening for admission: neurotic depressions, anxiety hysteria and phobias, sexual difficulty, character neuroses, and three cases of psychosis (who were transferred to the Psychotherapy Clinic). The average duration of clinic treatment was 320 hours per patient, with a range of from four months (a psychotic patient) to forty-two months. Only seven cases were of less than a year's duration; the others were treated for from one to three and a half years. Few cases completed their analyses in the clinic setting, the duration being from twenty-seven to thirty-nine months respectively.

In summary, we would like to re-emphasize our feeling that it would be of value in the very near future to have a report of a fairly extensive experience with the psychoanalytic therapy of patients in a clinic setting where no fee or a low fee is paid. In the light of the ever-growing tendency toward the integration of psychoanalysis with a university and with the former's multiple functioning in the teaching of medical students, the postgraduate instruction of residents and staff, as well as training them to do psychoanalytic therapy, will necessitate establishing psychoanalytic clinics where a larger number of patients can receive psychoanalytic therapy. This is indispensable because clinic work is a most important function in the training of psychoanalytic candidates. These clinics could very well be (and perhaps they should be) free clinics.

We may again think of Freud's words:

> . . . It may be a long time before the State regards this as an urgent duty. Present conditions may delay its arrival even longer; probably these institutions will first be started by private beneficence; some time or other, however, it must come.

It may be that the time has now come to consider seriously the establishment of clinics where psychoanalytic treatment can be offered without charge or for a very modest charge to those in need and without means. At this State University we have made a start.

REFERENCES

1. Bibring, E. The Mechanism of Depression. In: *Affective Disorders*, ed. P. Greenacre. New York: International Universities Press, 1953.
2. Deutsch, H. *The Psychology of Women*, 2 Vols. New York: Grune & Stratton, 1944, 1945.
3. Jones, E. The Early Development of Female Sexuality. *Papers on Psychoanalysis.* Baltimore: William & Wilkins, 1948.
4. Nunberg, H. The Will to Recovery. In: *Practice and Theory of Psychoanalysis*. New York: International Universities Press, 1955.

13

BRADFORD WILSON

I'm Not Getting Any Better

Second only to announcements of suicidal or homicidal intent, the phrase "I'm not getting any better," is perhaps the most unsettling that an analyst hears from a patient. That the literature on therapeutic technique abounds with vigorous rationales for dealing with this assertion merely underscores the sense of personal threat that it elicits in the bosom of the practicing psychotherapist.[1] Let us begin, by all means, with the candid admission that as professional persons who take our work seriously and are concerned with the therapeutic interaction rather than the mere execution of technical ploys, we *do care* about the patient's well-being and we *are concerned* when he asserts that his condition is not improving under our ministrations. Simply to dismiss the patient's complaint as a "nasty dig" at the therapist, or to treat it as an instance of infantile blame-shifting is both an insult to the patient and an abrogation of our therapeutic responsibility to examine our own behavior, techniques, and (most important of all) the underlying assumptions and attitudes that we bring to our interactions with a particular patient.

The chief goal of long-term psychotherapy is the attainment of

1. I use the terms psychoanalysis, analysis, psychotherapy, and therapy interchangeably. This is because I find that the distinctions commonly made between these words are not very useful. In the sense in which I use them, all aim at maximum insight, integration, and productive functioning of the total personality. Hence definitions based on whether the patient lies down/sits up, free-associates/controlled-associates, works/doesn't work with dreams, comes five times per week/once per week are really beside the point. Furthermore, the bulk of research into the matter strongly indicates that therapeutic success derives mainly from the personality and experience of the therapist, and not from the methods used.

insights and understandings that will eventually bear fruit in the form of more productive living. "The whole point of awareness is to avoid living out absurd destinies," says Allen Wheelis. I would add that to live out a misguided therapeutic interaction is as absurd a destiny as one can imagine, and one that can have far-flung and tragic consequences for the patient.[2]

From this it follows that the prime task for any therapist confronted with a patient who says he "is not getting any better" is to explore with utmost candor and honesty (in his own thinking and associations) not only the patient's possible reasons for saying it, but also his own manifold reactions to it. With this focus of discourse, let us undertake to examine some of the things that *might* be going on when a patient makes his unhappy assertion, keeping in mind that the therapist's manner of dealing with it depends largely upon the kind of construction he has placed on it. Beyond that, his handling of the matter comes under the heading of "personal style"—that intangible ingredient that evolves from the various Adaptation Levels[3] acquired from experiencing numerous therapeutic interactions.

Following are ten translations that may underly the statement "I'm not getting any better," together with a discussion of some of the dynamics that may be involved in each instance.

"I am literally drowning in my own material and am in more pain now than I ever was before."

From time to time in the course of therapy, a patient may bring up too much too quickly so that he becomes mired in his own analytic material. This is particularly liable to occur when volatile or highly sensitized patients are encouraged to lie down and free-associate. At other times the therapist may be overly eager to "get things onto the table," mistakenly viewing the patient's excess of zeal as an indication that the material "is ready to come up; otherwise it would remain safely repressed." In other words, a kind of *operant conditioning*[4] may be occurring in the therapeutic inter-

2. Some schools of psychoanalytic thought hold that a "well-analyzed" therapist should not even *have* (counter-transference) reactions to his patients in the *first* place, and maintain that if he *does*, he should remove himself from active practice and go back to "complete" his personal analysis—the underlying assumption (*pre*sumption would be a better word) being that a well-analyzed therapist never espouses an erroneous viewpoint, and has no risidual conflicts or distortions; in short, that he is *incapable of error*.

3. Helson defines *Adaptation Level* as a process whereby "organisms pool incoming impulses from focal and background stimuli with residuals from past experience to form adaptation levels, which in turn are *weighted averages* of these three classes of stimuli."

4. Operant conditioning, as defined and extensively used by Skinner in his

action whereby the patient is being subtly induced to regurgitate more and more "analytic material"—perhaps to assuage the therapist's doubts about his own competence (for it happens most often with beginning therapists), or to satisfy various other needs.

One young woman likened the experience of being swamped to "a blob—a helpless baby lying in a dirty diaper while the mess builds up, and wishing somebody would help me to *deal* with it." This patient was in fact saying "You *allowed* me to overproduce; now don't just *sit* there, *do* something!" And she was right. When I stopped to reflect that her babyhood took place during the "Let 'em Cry" era of child-rearing,[5] I realized that a stoical "I-shall-not-cater-to-the-patient's-demand-for-a-'magic-helper' " response on my part would be not only cruel and irresponsible (after all, I had indeed helped her into the mess), but would also constitute an unbearable recapitulation of the sort of emotional neglect that lay at the root of her adult helplessness. While some schools of analytic persuasion let the patients "cry themselves out" under such circumstances, it seems doubtful whether the strength gained does much toward solving the interactional challenge whereby the patient who has grown up in a seemingly indifferent world may now learn that he can sometimes hold others accountable for *their* share of the responsibility and can ask for and receive redress of grievances.

Given the correctness of the translation as offered, the easiest method for handling the situation is to share the foregoing insights with the patient in whatever manner seems appropriate.

"Tell me it isn't true. I don't really know what is going on here, and life has taught me to assume the worst. I need information."

There are two basic approaches to psychotherapy, and while they are not mutually exclusive, therapists tend to lean more heavily toward one or the other. In the first, coming down to us through Freud and his followers, the therapist seeks to "confront" the patient with his own distorted and regressed ways of dealing with the world. This involves, more often than not, the automatic withholding of any and all responses that are (or seem to be) "demanded" by the patient. The second approach was first expounded by Ferenczi and is grounded in the assumption that most (if not all) of the patient's difficulties arise out of distorted "lessons" learned in a distorted

---

experiments with animals, is to be distinguished from classical (stimulus-response or Pavlovian that) conditioning by virtue of the fact that it involves the reinforcement of behaviors which *emerge spontaneously from the organism's natural repertoire*—rather than being placed there by external means.

5. This attitude was in vogue during the 1920's and 30's in America. Mothers were encouraged to let their infants cry untended whenever possible in order to discourage "excessive dependency."

environment. For this reason the therapist must now provide for the patient a number of *new* and *un*distorted experiences from which the patient may derive new and undistorted lessons.

It might be useful for the therapist to ask himself whether a beneficial experience for the patient might be accomplished by simply extending a supportive hand, as it were, by saying something such as, "You *are* getting better; actually, you're doing fine! Look how you have been able to do this, and that, and the other–things you could never have done a year or even six months ago." The time-honored technique of "tossing the question back into the patient's lap" would be of limited value here. Some patients have never gotten a pat on the back for anything they have done, so that a kind word from the therapist now and then can often accomplish more than several years of Spartan self-confrontation.

It should be added that in the lives of many patients their childhood questions were ignored altogether, or else only partially or inappropriately responded to. Thus, questions about progress in therapy (and other questions as well) may represent an attempt in later life to rebuild the shattered communication bridge of childhood. It does not, of course, necessitate a constant answering of questions on the therapist's part, only an open acknowledgment of the *right to ask them*. In this way we make possible more productive communication and feedback.

"I'm about to undertake some new and frightening challenges; if I were still as mixed up as I used to be, I'd never have gotten myself into this new mess. Tell me I'm not ready for it yet."

Like an animal about to scale a high wall, the psyche often steps back a number of paces and crouches down, as it were, ready to spring forward. This may result in the phenomenological experience of standing still or going backwards. By exploring the possibility of new undertakings on the part of the patient (which may as yet be only in the planning stages), a perspective may be gained that can bring with it the kind of relief one feels when an optical illusion is satisfactorily explained. Possible reasons underlying the fear of new challenges will be discussed in later sections of this paper.

"I've done my part in putting in my time here. Why hasn't the Great Miracle taken place?"

It is axiomatic that people seek help for their emotional problems not out of any wish to change their way of doing things, but rather from a persistent and tireless hope that the analyst will take their unsuccessful techniques and somehow transform them into useful tools for living. A pet dog of mine, who dearly loved motor trips, would occasionally sneak into the car where he would place himself squarely behind the driver's seat. There he would sit, sometimes for an hour at a stretch, apparently waiting for the vehicle to begin moving. Patients in psychotherapy can sometimes do the same thing. This is particularly true among catatonic-like individuals, whom somebody has described as "suffering from a strangulation of volition." These people need a certain amount of firm but judicious *prodding* or they may immobilize their lives indefinitely, and their statement, "I'm not getting any better," will represent an accurate appraisal of their situation.

A therapist working with this type of patient must ask himself whether he, too, is perhaps indulging in the same kind of assumption, for example, that as long as the patient continues to pay his fee and to appear regularly for sessions, something must eventually "give." If so, it *may* be an example of operant conditioning from *patient* to *therapist*, rather than from therapist to patient. It must also be conceded that a certain amount of fatalism is inevitable, considering how limited is our present knowledge of why some patients progress in therapy while others do not. However, the danger inherent in such fatalistic thinking lies in its potential for producing an ever more rarified therapeutic atmosphere in which the interaction becomes less and less relevant to the patient's daily life. For as the balloon of the therapy ascends higher and higher into a sort of do-nothing stratosphere, one finds that less and less is taking place on "terra firma," in the daily life of the patient.

"I still don't feel comfortable about coming here. All we do is rake up garbage; there's never any fun in it."

Some people enter psychotherapy with such eagerness to be good patients that they rush about like distracted puppies, sniffing into every corner of their newfound psyche and dragging out an incredible assortment of old bones, tattered slippers, stale biscuits, and "dust feathers" in their all-out efforts to win the approval of the therapist.

It is in this connection that the most virulent form of mutually operant conditioning in psychotherapy takes place, for it is an unhappy fact that many patients (and therapists as well) have the misguided notion that they are "not analyzing" unless a Platter of Worms is served up at each and every session. This devolves largely from the problem-centered viewpoint of our clinical tradition that tends to regard psychotherapy solely as a "treatment" situation aimed at the relentless pursuit of problems and conflicts, rather than the more inclusive goal of also helping patients to contact and realize their own capacities for pleasure and self-fulfillment. Because the same attitude afflicts lay conceptions of psychoanalysis, the patient usually drags these problem-centered assumptions with him into the therapy, where they may go undetected by a therapist who is already inclined to regard the patient as "very disturbed"[6] and therefore *expecting* (conditioning?) each session to be rife with symptoms, conflicts, and reports of aberrant behavior.

The therapist, then, may need to explore his *own* attitudes about playing and having fun. Has the child (in himself or in the patient) somehow become *outlawed* in the zealous quest for emotional maturity and social adulthood? Lawrence K. Frank has pointed out the enormous value of (judicious) parental participation in a child's play life and its affects upon the development of reality-testing. The same principles have applicability in therapy, for what else are we doing if not raising children, in a certain sense? That which is already mature, growing, and functioning in the patient needs no *help* from us, although it certainly does need our affirmation. But it is the *damaged child* in the patient who most needs our help and encouragement.

Nowhere is the necessity for *learning how to play* more evident than it is in some schizophrenic and most schizoid persons. Rado has noted the wide prevalence of "anhedonia" in schizophrenic patients, and Meehl considers it pathognomonic. We need to explore, in our own behavior, the degree to which we may be confirming (and even encouraging) so gloomy a *weltanschauung*. Anyone who has observed a student therapist greeting his patients in a clinic setting is not likely to forget the "Life is real; life is earnest" quality of the interaction—conducted like a sombre pavane in which both the participants behave more like cellmates in Death Row than partners in an adventurous quest for self-knowledge. I have even known more experienced colleagues to behave that way over luncheon, no less!

When I speak of "play" in the therapeutic interaction, I certainly don't mean that the therapy should be converted into a Laugh-in or an opera buffa. But someone once defined humor as "an awareness of the contrast between things as they *ought* to be and things as they *are*." It is precisely this awareness that can produce a kind of playfulness in therapy that I have found to be highly beneficial, especially with patients who tend to be either too vulnerable, or overly excitable, or both. Such an approach is counterindicated when dealing with patients whose character disorders tend to make a certain kind of impertinent humor their stock in trade. Humor should never be used for purposes of watering down or avoiding intense feelings, and the therapist should be careful that the attempted humor doesn't fit into a patient's tendency to *self*-ridicule.

One way of righting a "gloom and doom" imbalance is to make a

6. Owing to the fact that patients usually come to us in times of dire trouble and crisis, we rarely see them with their best foot forward. Hence, it is all too easy for us to forget, sometimes, that there may be a number of areas in their life pictures wherein their functioning is not only adequate but even *superb*.

remark such as, "I notice the things you've been bringing in here have been exclusively *unpleasant*; I wonder why that is.... does *nothing good* ever happen to you?" This almost invariably leads to the patient's revealing his notion that reporting happy events is taboo in psychotherapy. ("That's not what we're *here* for, is it? I didn't think you'd be interested. I'm supposed to talk about my problems.") Or, it may lead to a discussion of "money's-worth" in therapy. ("I'm paying money to solve my *problems*—why waste time talking about the *happy* things?") In either case, the only therapeutic answer, in my opinion, is to point out that the analytic collaboration involves *all* aspects of the personality and of living, not just a single perspective.

"I'm really getting better, but you (like everybody else in this dog-eat-dog world) will cut me down if I let you know it. Or else you'll assign me a new and bigger task that I'm not ready for yet."

Some people grow up in an environment where there always seemed to be a penalty connected with any sense of accomplishment or well-being the individual managed to achieve. Retribution invariably appeared in the shape of a rivalrous sibling, a competitive adult, or whatever. The result is usually the superstitious conviction that happiness is a punishable offense that invites terrible and swift retaliation from unknown quarters. I don't know how much truth there is to it, but I have been told that Jerusalem's famous Wailing Wall, contrary to popular opinion, is *not* a place where the devout go to bemoan their *misfortunes*; rather it is a place where people go in times of *prosperity*, hoping by their histrionic protestations of misery to avert future calcmity at the hands of their jealous God. Similarly, patients in psychoanalysis may utilize a Wailing Wall technique for staving off an anticipated disaster. According to George Kelly, most—if not all—of human behavior is based upon the constructs whereby each of us anticipates future happenings.

The maintenance of weakness and suffering—often called Masochism—may represent a "playing possum" strategy aimed at throwing potential predators off the scent. A woman who had been obese throughout her adult life put it quite succinctly: "After all, who's going to attack me as long as I remain a fat, ugly mess?"[7]

Some patients grew up with parents who were deeply disappointed or inadequate persons and who conveyed the notion that any self-fulfillment on the part of their offspring represented food snatched from their own hungry mouths. This is especially characteristic of depressive mothers who tend to regard any jollity as a personal

7. So acute is the anxiety experienced by many obese persons who lose large quantities of weight (through crash-dieting procedures and such-like) that they do not feel safe until they have regained it *all*.

affront to their own suffering. The children of such parents usually come to treat pleasure and self-fulfillment as loaded weapons that they tinker with at their own peril. Going hand-in-hand with this is the child's reluctance to let himself rise above the stature of his parents; if he cannot see them as truly "big" people, he can at least make them *seem* bigger by making himself *smaller*. "I'm not getting any better" is one way of doing this.

There are also those parents who seize on the child's every accomplishment as an excuse for setting up ever larger tasks for him to fulfill. "Now that you know how to make your own bed, maybe you can start cooking your own meals." A parent eager to escape the burdens of parenthood is particularly adept at this. What it means for the patient is that each and every move toward increased independence and self-sufficiency is experienced as yet another step along the road to orphanhood. And who in this world would willingly choose to be an orphan?

The therapist confronted with this kind of maneuver does well to ask himself whether anything in the interaction has given the patient *reason* to believe that his accomplishments will somehow be "punished" by the therapist. Sometimes a raise in fee which follows too closely on the heels of a patient's job promotion can convey such an impression.[8] Or, perhaps the therapist has been too eager to rush the patient on to bigger and better things, for there are some therapists who gauge their own professional success by the public accomplishments of their patients.

"In my capacity to endure suffering lies my greatest strength; you shall not deprive me of it!"

For many people, both in and out of psychotherapy, the greatest success story of their entire biography is the fact that they managed, by sheer endurance, to survive their childhood. And by the looks of it, this is no mean accomplishment! However, for many persons the mere act of suffering can take on *tool* properties so that in time of stress they reach for their "trusty weapon," often seeking out ways and means by which to bring about their own agony and ensure ultimate victory. "Suffering," proclaimed one patient "is the incantation I use to produce victory in the final analysis—no pun intended." Another said "I don't want to die in my sleep, I want to know in advance so that I can suffer; then maybe I can escape death altogether!"

Given the patient's assumption that his suffering has survival value,

8. Needless to say, sudden raises in fee are sometimes unavoidable,—as for example when a patient who has been seen for a clinic fee suddenly reveals that his net annual income is twice that of the therapist, whereupon the fee is—(or *should* be)—promptly and unceremoniously hiked.

the amelioration of it can be a most frightening experience until such time as its tool properties are replaced by a sense of having other instrumentalities at his disposal. As a matter of fact, he may have already acquired them but is not yet aware of the fact—in which case it would be a good idea for the therapist to point it out for him. Again, psychoanalysis should include the interpretation of the patient's strengths as well as his limitations. In this instance, the patient needs some reassurance that it is safe not to suffer.

"You are the first person to take an interest in me and to care about me; maybe I'd better quit while I'm ahead."

Here the patient expresses his underlying fear that if the therapist gets to know "the real me," he will toss him out on his ear. Every session, then, seems to be bringing him closer to his own inevitable exile. Thus the complaint, "I'm not getting any better," while couched in the form of a *prophesy*, actually represents a statement of *intention*. It is an intention to forestall the dreaded insight by marking time and in that way bringing the ongoing process of psychotherapy to a standstill.

There may have been one or several severe losses of some beloved person in the patient's life, and in this case the formula becomes, "Every time I begin to feel accepted and safe in a relationship, the person dies or goes away; I am abandoned." With patients who have a history of desertion special care should be taken to see that they receive postcards from the therapist during summer vacations or other periods of prolonged absence.[9]

Such patients are particularly convinced that the therapist never gives them a thought outside of sessions. The ego-psychologists point to the importance of this factor in the early formation of the child's self-concept: When the child is able to believe that the absent mother carries him *lovingly in her thoughts*, a positive self-image results; otherwise the self comes to be regarded as garbage or "throw-away" material.

The therapeutic interaction should be examined in an effort to discover whether the therapist may have inadvertently provided grounds for the patient's fears. For example, has he forgotten some appointments with this patient? (Forgetting an appointment can happen even to the most experienced of us.) Have some vacation postcards gone astray? Did he insufficiently prepare the patient for a long absence? Was an appointment suddenly cancelled? Did the therapist accidentally "double up" an appointment and give the hour to another patient in the presence of this one? Has the therapist been

9. I am reminded of one patient who had experienced no less that *eight* major losses by the age of seven, and who invariably took to his bed like a sick animal whenever the therapist was away for an extended period.

in ill health recently? (Schizophrenic patients are especially sensitive to any weakening of the analyst's physical stamina, and their reactions to it are often catastrophic.)

I do not believe that patients pull their anticipations entirely out of thin air. More often than not the therapist has done something, albeit in the standard routine of his work, that has *triggered* certain predispositions on the part of the patient. The assumption that patients are invariably *eliciting* negative behaviors from the analyst is open to considerable question. The fact that a patient may *expect* a dreary kind of experience does not necessarily imply that he is setting it up single-handedly. Much unwarranted difficulty—and perhaps the therapy itself—can be saved by stopping now and then to survey what has or has not transpired in the therapeutic interaction.

"I am suffering, and if you really cared you would make it go away, then I could believe that I am lovable."

As infants, we have the inherent right to expect that our biological mother will sense our needs without our having to spell them out and administer to them. Unfortunately, some mothers are unable to fulfill this function, so the child is faced with the terrible question of *why* he is being so neglected or mistreated. As a helpless toddler in a world of "giants" upon whom he depends for his very existence, he dare not conclude that his guardians are weak, limited, or irrational; hence the only alternative is to conclude, "It must be *me*; something must be wrong with me; I am not lovable enough." Added to this, he includes the full weight of his punctured infantile grandiosity that says in effect, "Since *you* are "magical," you *could*, if you wanted to, spare me all pain and grant me any wish under the sun. But you do neither, obviously because I am not lovable enough."

The individual's major quest in life becomes the search for the perfect love—that benign giant who will banish care and fulfill dreams, and by so doing prove to the individual's satisfaction that he is indeed lovable.

As therapists, we are trained from the outset to be aware of these strivings on the part of patients and to guard against them at all costs. We are warned against the dangers of "playing God," and admonished not to do anything that might encourage fantasies of a grandiose or in ordinately demanding nature. While none can cavil with the wisdom of such advice, it does seem to me that we may lean too far over in the opposite direction: "Why *should* I?" retorts one analyst to a patient who accuses him of not caring, "Do you have to be heard *all* the time?" demands another when a patient accuses her of not listening. In short, it is an all-too-common practice to dismiss all reaching out for affirmation or support on the part of the patient as mere manifestations of the inordinate and gargantuan demands that troubled persons are wont to impose on their environments. Yet if we look back upon our own personal analysis (provided it was a bona fide therapy experience), we will surely recall times when we were genuinely downhearted and in need of encouragement. If our own therapist made the mistake of treating the situation callously, that is no justification for us to do so with our *own* patients. We do well if we can profit from our own therapist's mistakes as well as from his strengths. The fact is that there are times when the patient needs *tenderness*, and if we are afraid to show our humanity, how can we ever help our patients to accept *theirs*? A colleague once told me that a turning point in her life came (after six years of "Let 'em Cry" therapy) when she proclaimed from the depths of her despair that nobody in the world cared whether she lived or died, and her new analyst said very simply, "*I* care."

We must ask ourselves whether, in our efforts to provide an "objective" atmosphere, we may sometimes extend our dispassion to a point where it is equivalent to cruelty. There is the realistic possibility that, much as we dislike admitting it, the patient may be correct—he really is *not* making any progress in the therapy.

This raises the uncomfortable issue of our own vanity as professional persons, for when confronted with a patient who is at a standstill, it is very tempting to conclude that he must be "untreatable." A more useful approach is to share with the patient the possibility that, for some intangible reason, our personalities may not be suited for further work together. The patient should be encouraged to air his views about the therapist candidly. Maybe some personal attributes or idiosyncracies of the therapist are setting off adverse reactions in the patient. Or perhaps there is some aspect of the therapy situation itself that is causing trouble. Following are some examples of dynamics that can be triggered in patients by the mere *mechanics* of psychotherapy:

Inequality — The patient is required to "tell all" about himself while the therapist reveals relatively little.[10] Patients from strict, rigid, old-fashioned, or authoritarian backgrounds are highly vulnerable to this aspect of psychotherapy. Children of attorneys are especially prone to view the situation as a painful recapitulation of the recurrent childhood scene in which they were subjected to one-sided, courtroom-like cross examinations without benefit of counsel. Such patients often enter therapy "claim-

10. In a *direct* way, that is,—for even the "mm-hmm" school of psychoanalysis reveals far more about the therapist than one would believe possible. If anything, it is the most powerful form of operant conditioning in use today.

ing the Fifth," and their progress in therapy may be severely hampered by their fear that what they reveal may one day be used by the therapist in some devious manner.

Prying

Some patients grew up in homes where the parents made a career of "taking an interest" in their children's activities. The children grew up in veritable goldfish bowls where parental eyes monitored their bedsheets, their underwear, their bathroom habits, and their personal relationships. As a result, these patients are acutely sensitive to any questioning or probing on the part of the therapist, no matter how understanding or compassionate. What these people need from the therapy, paradoxically enough, is respect for their *privacy*—which is, of course, the exact antithesis of psychotherapy as most practitioners regard it. Yet if the prerogative *not to reveal* isn't openly acknowledged at the outset, these patients are unlikely to surmount the serious problem presented to them by the very nature of the therapy situation.

Discussing Family Matters

Many children—especially those from families that had a good deal to hide—are indoctrinated from their earliest years not to reveal family business to "strangers." Doing so constitutes the height of perfidy. Yet now they are being asked in their analysis to "tell *all*." Many of these patients would rather completely reject the therapy and the therapist than commit such an act of "treason" against the secrecy of the family.

Complaining

There is a type of parent who feels particularly helpless when his child is in pain. In his desperate efforts to alleviate the distress he may turn upon the pain itself and "punish" it by putting an instant stop to all tears, all whining, all expressions of distress. The methods for doing this are often quite severe and may include corporal punishment, being sent to bed without food, castor oil spread on a slice of bread—with the result that built-in prohibitions against complaining can exert a powerful counterpull to the cathartic inducements of the therapy situation.

The Fee

As we well know, many patients regard the fee as an impersonal transaction that vitiates the intimacy of the therapeutic relationship. For the lonely or isolated patient, it is often a devastating experience to find himself in a position where the only person who gives him any attention is being *paid* to do so. I have found it helpful to point out that, while necessity dictates that I be paid for my work, I still hold the prerogative of determining the patients with whom I wish, or do *not* wish, to work.

Time of Day Some patients "work better" in the early morning or late morning or early afternoon or evening. Schizophrenics and other persons who tend to be overwhelmed by the day's events work much better shortly after they awaken. The difference between a morning and an evening session for them can sometimes be extraordinary. In the evening they may be so shattered that it takes the entire session to pick up the pieces, whereas in the morning these same people are likely to be serene, communicative, open to insight, and more sanguine in their view of life.

While it is obvious that most of the foregoing obstacles represent inherent, and for the most part unmodifiable, aspects of the therapy situation per se, there is merit in airing such issues in the therapeutic interaction. It may otherwise be helpful to suggest to the patient that he try seeing another therapist once a week "while continuing our own work as usual until we find out how the wind is blowing." In this way we avoid any action that might imply that we are punishing the patient for "not getting well." Unceremoniously dismissing the patient would certainly justify such an interpretation. In point of fact, I have found no harm and much benefit from having some patients work with a second therapist on a regular basis. Fears that the patient will "play off" one therapist against the other turn out to be almost entirely unfounded.

"I have endured the humiliation of letting you witness my many failings; now I will get even by proving you to be the biggest failure of all!"

This, of course, is the classical "negative transference" construction that therapists of all persuasions probably place on the statement "I'm not getting any better." It is known to be the favorite maneuver of chronically depressed persons, as can be attested to by anyone who has worked with them therapeutically—or known them *socially*, for that matter.

I have placed it last on the list because I think it should be resorted to *only* when all other possibilities have been carefully explored and ruled out. Further discussion of this translation can be found in almost any textbook on psychoanalytic technique.

In conclusion, the foregoing has been a discussion of *some* of the dynamics that may underly the common complaint of patients, "I'm not getting any better." To interpret the patient's dynamics solely in terms of a distorted projection upon the so-called "blank screen" of the therapist's "incognito" is, I think, to ignore the maxim that no one projects onto thin air: For example, the proverbial spinster does not choose an asexual man on whom to project her rape fantasies. Likewise, there is more often than not a certain validity to the patient's projections upon the therapist, however exaggerated may be their final manifestation. For the therapist to exempt from scrutiny his own role in the therapeutic interaction is not only negligent and arrogant, but a highly destructive form of self-indulgence as well. Psychotherapy is at its best when it constitutes a voyage of self-discovery, not only for the patient, but also for the analyst.

REFERENCES

1. Frank, L. K. "Play in Personality Development," in *The Child*, Jerome Seidman, New York: Rinehart & Co. Inc., 1958.
2. Helson, H. "Some Problems in Motivation From the Point of View of Adaptation Level." *Nebraska Symposium on Motivation,* University of Nebraska Press, 1966.
3. Kelley, G. *The Psychology of Personal Contructs*, New York: W. W. Norton & Co., 1955.
4. Meehl, P. E. "Schizotaxia, Schizopyty, Schizophrenia," *American Psychologist* 1962, 17, 827-838.
5. Rado, S. *Psychoanalysis of Behavior*, New York: Grune & Stratton, 1956.
6. Weil, E. "The Origin and Visissitudes of the Self Image," *Psychoanalysis,* 1958, 6 (1).
7. Wheelis A. *The Seeker,* New York: Random House, 1959.

14

SHELDON B. KOPP

The Refusal to Mourn

> There are two kinds of sorrow . . . When a man broods over the misfortunes that have come upon him, when he cowers in a corner and despairs of help—that is a bad kind of sorrow . . . The other kind is the honest grief of a man whose house has burned down, who feels his need deep in his soul and begins to build anew.[1]

To some extent each of us still lives in the darkness of his own unfinished past. The refusal to mourn the disappointments and losses of childhood, to bury them once and for all, condemns us to live in their shadows.[2] Genuine grief is the sobbing and wailing that express the acceptance of our helplessness to do anything about losses. If instead, we whine and complain, insist that this cannot be, or demand to be compensated for our pain, then we are forever stuck with trying to redeem the past.

In some ways, psychotherapy is basically a difficult moral venture. It is the attempt by the therapist to help the patient to become and to live as a decent human being, no matter how hard a time he has had. He must learn to live well, in the present, beginning with things as they are and open to the ambiguities of this mixed bag of a world as it is. And all of this he must do in spite of the fact that he has been cheated; has had to stand by helplessly while he was ignored, betrayed, undone; while he watched his hopes shattered, his most precious possessions lost, and his dreams unrealized. What is more, if he refuses to accept the misfortunes of the past as unalterable, then he does not get to keep the warm loved feelings intact. These joys of yesterday and of now will be open to being somehow spoiled whenever he feels helpless about some new loss.

Or perhaps there *are* only different kinds of unhappy childhoods,

1. Hasidic saying from Martin Buber, *Tales of the Hasidism: The Early Masters*, New York, Schocken Books, 1966, p. 231.
2. Robert J. Wetmore, "The Role of Grief in Psycho-Analysis," *International Journal of Psycho-Analysis*, Vol. 44, Part 1, 1963, pp. 97-103.

and remembrances of happy childhoods are merely illusions, desperately held on to. Children are, after all, inevitably helpless and dependent, no matter what resources they may develop for coping with that towering world in which they live. Parents always turn out to be a disappointment, one way or another. Frustrations are many, and life is inherently unmanageable. "Momma may have, Poppa may have, but God bless the child that's got his own, that's got his own."[3]

As children, we all really are helpless to change our worlds, or to move on and take care of ourselves when we cannot. Unable to give up hope on such a life-and-death matter, the child is confronted with the desperate anxiety that Farber describes as resulting from trying to will that which cannot be willed.[4] Each child finds ways of pretending to himself that he is not as powerless as he feels. He must maintain the illusion that somehow he can get his parents to love him as he wishes to be loved. Panic over his helplessness must be transformed into a stubborn struggle to get his own way, even if only in fantasy. The more he has been treated as though his feelings did not count, the greater his own resultant willfulness. It is in the service of maintaining the illusion that he can get his own way, that his neurotic behavior is endlessly and irreleventry repeated and that self-restricting risk-avoiding character styles develop.

In this way, to varying degrees, do people insist that the world has to be fair, that they must either get what they want or someone must pay. Thus, for example:

> An obsessively worried young man points out that he can never be happy, never really free to enjoy his successes, because he was raised by so mean and selfish a father, and so undependably vague a mother. His suffering is their indictment and he won't let them off the hook.
>
> An hysterical young woman insists that since she has had to put up with disappointments in the past, certainly by now some wonderful person must come along and take care of her.
>
> Another tells us of what a very awful person she is. It is not that mother was selfish or unloving, but rather just that even as a little girl she was too bad abnormal, or somehow unsatisfactory to warrant better treatment. And now if she can only improve enough, things with Momma would/have, could/have, will be different.
>
> Yet another fellow goes the opposite route, showing how little he needs others, how uncaring and above it all he is. If only he had good Le Bret, that

3. Arthur Herzog, Jr. and Billie Holiday, *God Bless' the Child*, Edward B. Marks Music Corporation, 1941.

4. Leslie Farber, "Will and Anxiety," *The Ways of the Will*, New York, Basic Books, 1966, pp. 26-50.

friend of Cyrano's to whisper to him: "Be proud and bitter, but underneath your breath—whisper 'she loves me not—and that is death.' "[5]

There are, of course, many and varied ways in which adults may continue to play out these childhood struggles. What they have in common is limited commitment to the meaning of their lives as it stands. Rather, their common outcry is: "I've been cheated and I won't stand for it. I must have my way. If not, at the very least, others will not get their way with me again." The adult in whom the unmet unmourned child dwells, stubbornly insists that he has the power to make someone love him, or else to make them feel sorry for not doing so. Appeasing, wheedling, bribing, or bullying are carried out in stubborn hope that if only he is submissive enough, sneaky enough, bad enough, upset enough, something enough . . . then he will get his own way.

Part of the therapist's task is to avoid getting entangled by the patient's attempts at emotional blackmail, intimidation, seductive adoration, dependent demands, and the like. Of course, the therapist is likely to be hooked into responding to these maneuvers in some ways, but then the recognition and disentangling get the patient to begin looking at what he is up to. The therapist tries to arouse the patient's curiousity about his own life. At the same time that the therapist is interrupting these self-defeating strategies, by not going along with them, he is also insisting on being recognized as a person in his own right, with feelings that count. He must find ways to let the patient know that:

> My pain hurts as yours does. Each of us has the same amount to lose, all we have. My tears are as bitter, my scars as permanent. My loneliness is an aching in my chest, much like yours. Who are you to feel that your losses mean more than mine. What arrogance! "I feel angry at your ignoring my feelings. I live in the same imperfect world in which you struggle, a world in which, like you, I must make do with less than I would wish for myself.
>
> And too, you seem to feel that you should be able to succeed without failure, to love without loss, to reach out without risk of disappointment, never to appear vulnerable or even foolish. . . . Why? While the rest of us must sometimes fall, be hurt, feel inadequate, but rise again and go on. Why do you feel that you alone should be spared all this? How did you become so special? In what way have you been chosen?
>
> You say you've had a bad time of it, an unhappy childhood? Me too. You say that you didn't get all you needed and wanted, weren't always understood or cared for? Welcome to the club.

The therapist must help the patient to see that for each of them,

5. Edmond Rostand, *Cyrano de Bergerac*, Mount Vernon, New York, Peter Pauper Press, 1941, Act II.

this session is an hour of his life, no more to be recaptured by the one then by the other. They could become important to one another, but only to the extent that each disarms himself, takes chances on being vulnerable to be hurt by the other, to risk new losses.

As the interaction focuses the patient's attention on past losses and on what he has to lose in the encounter with the therapist, he must be left no quarter. He can only keep what he really had. When he insists that his parents loved him "in their own way," he must be faced with the realization that this is an inference. When parental love is offered in a form that is negotiable, when it is directed toward how the child feels, then it can be experienced directly by the child. It does not need to be inferred. And to the extent that the patient did not get what he wanted or needed or was entitled to, simply because he was their kid, that's rough, but that's it.

All he can do now is to try to face how really bad he feels, and how stuck he is with it. Then he may turn to others in his life, and try to be open enough so that they may get to know him. He can make his wishes known, and if they come through, fine. If not, if they know him but they don't love him, then there's nothing to be done about it. Perhaps someone else will love him. But in any case, no one can take anyone else's place. It will never be made up to him. He will just have to do without, like it or not, and face his losses and his helplessness to change them. He must weep, and mourn and grieve them through. He must unhook from the past to make room for the present. In burying the parents of childhood, he must make do with the rest of the world minus two. Not such a bad trade after all.

By no longer refusing to mourn the loss of the parents whom he wished for but never had, he can get to keep whatever was really there for him. He may come to know that not getting his own way does not always mean he is not loved. No longer living in the seemingly ordered world of childhood, in which good and suffering are supposed to be rewarded, and evil and selfishness punished, he must nonetheless try to do his best to live decently. An unhappy childhood is not a justification for copping out. Life is a mixed bag, at best, for everyone. Each man must face disappointment, frustration, failure, loss and betrayal, illness, aging, and finally his own death. And yet, he must face up to Camus' challenge: *To be a just man in an unjust world.*[6] To find life arbitrary, and yet to take things as they are, to bring to them what you can, and to enjoy them as they stand, because this is it; often unsatisfying, at times dis-

6. Albert Camus, "Letters to a German Friend," *Resistance, Rebellion and Death*, New York, The Modern Library, 1960, pp. 3-25.

appointing, always imperfect. But it's the only world we have . . . .Can you be loving in it, and bring to it the meaning of your own being and willingness. Can you live without illusions in a world where there is no appeal?[7] Can you love in the absence of illusions?

To take up this challenge, deceptively simple insights, too fundamental to be grasped once and for all, must be learned, not just once, but renewed again and again. As Hemingway tells us: "There are some things which cannot be learned quickly and time, which is all we have, must be paid heavily for their acquiring."[8] As though it were not enough to struggle with the arbitrary parameters of childhood, once free of them, each man must realize other elusive truths such as: Each of us is, in his own terms, vulnerable. Each is as weak and as strong as the other, as tough and as tender, as capable of good and of evil, and consequently, each is as fully responsible for his actions as the other. And too, that it is so very exciting and so terribly hard to be a grown-up human being (perhaps almost as hard as it is to be a child).

As a grown-up, *ultimately each man is alone*. No one can do for him what he must do for himself. You got to walk that lonesome valley, "You got to walk it by yourself, nobody else can walk it for you, you got to walk it by yourself."[9] No other's solution will do. Each man has to contend with the same fundamental condition of being *here*, and *now*, and *himself and no other*. Yet for each it is different, even while being the same. It differs mainly in that I am not you, though our plight is the same.

Each man's relation to every other man is ironically drawn in Samuel Beckett's novel, *Molloy*.[10] This two-part tale begins by telling of Molloy, the anti-hero: a dirty, unkempt, snot-dripper; a crippled, festering, rag-clad derilect, wandering without purpose; a scatological consciousness and a social shamble. His journey in exile reduces him still further, till he is no longer simply misfit, degenerate, and outcast, but also put upon, beaten and almost killed. Even his crutches are of little use when he ends up alone, still homeless, and now exausted, barely managing to crawl through the snowy forest night toward the light of the plains far in the distance, perhaps toward shelter, warmth, or maybe even home.

The second part of the novel tells of Moran, a man of consequence who is (and has) everything Molloy is not. He has a home and family,

7. Albert Camus, "An Absurd Reasoning," *The Myth of Sisyphus, and Other Essays*, New York, Vintage Books, 1960, pp. 3-48.
8. Ernest Hemmingway, *Death in the Afternoon*, New York, Charles Scribner's Sons, 1932, p. 192.
9. Anonymous, *Lonesome Valley*, Spiritual in Public Domain.
10. Samuel Beckett, *Molloy*, New York, Grove Press, 1955.

a place in the church and in the community. He is clean, well-tailored, barbered and manicured, altogether well turned out. He also has an assignment: "Get Molloy." Without knowing just why or on whose orders, he sets out to see about fulfilling this obligation. He is never sure whether he has found him, though it may in fact have been Molloy whom he at one point beat and almost killed. But in his pursuit of Molloy, Moran ends up losing his way, is separated from his family and his position, is attacked and injured so that he must use his umbrella as a crutch. And finally, unshaven, uncombed, unwashed and hungry, his clothes in tatters, he ends up alone, homeless and exausted, barely managing to crawl through the freezing night rain, toward a house far in the distance, which he hopes will provide shelter, warmth, or maybe even home.

Thus, we had best come to know one another, for there is little else for us in this world. We must each learn what it is we have to give to the other, and what it is we may hope to receive. It is so very hard sometimes to be a human being: a grown-up, limited, at times helpless, take-care-of-yourself-cause-no-one-else-will individual person. What can we hope to be for one another in this frightening, exciting world in which we are both free and trapped? What I hope to give to my patients–as well as what I also hope to get from my patients–is the courage and comfort of knowing someone else who faces his life as it is, risks the knowing, feels what I feel, struggles as I struggle, mourns his losses–and survives.

We must live, I believe, in the face of knowing that man is, ultimately, not perfectable. Evil can be redistributed but never eradicated. Each solution creates new problems, and the temptation to cop out is ever present. Perhaps all that we can hope for is to be committed to the struggle to do our best as much as we are able. And the relationship between patient and therapist, between man and man, is a community of sinners. Loving and joyful though we may sometimes be, "the wish to kill is never killed, but with some gift of courage one may look into its face when it appears, and with a stroke of love–as to an idiot in the house–forgive it; again and again . . . forever."[11]

By mourning our losses and burying our dead, in therapy, and in the rest of life, we open ourselves to the only real contact we can have with others . . .touching now, standing in the rubble of the past. For *we are all Jews.*[12] We all wander in exile. We suffer, trying to believe that there is a reason. We try to go our way and to do what is right. But at times each of us forgets that we are all Jews. We want

11. Arthur Miller, *After the Fall*, New York, Viking Press, 1964, Act II.
12. This concept was developed in dialogue with Dr. Vincent O'Connell at an American Academy of Psychotherapists Workshop in June, 1968.

some certainty, some clarity. We want the face of the enemy at last to be clear and for the good guys to win once and for all. At that point, when any man forgets that he is a Jew, denies that he is in exile, at that point he runs the risk of becoming a Nazi. In his quest for home, for permanence, for clarity and dependable meaning, he may define himself by becoming the one who defines others; defines them as Jews by persecuting them, or more insidiously, by separating himself from them, by denying their common humanity.

Our only hope is as a community of exiles. Wanderers, wherever they are from, are Jews, whatever their religion. Exiles from the illusions of childhood, the illusion of the all-good family and of the certain place in a world that makes sense. It matters not whether a man is self-exiled in response to disappointment and in search of a more meaningful place, a promised land; or if for another man, the original comforting illusion was violently wrenched away. What matters is that *the loss of innocence is permanent*. There is no returning. There is only the community of wanderers, the touching of hands by passing exiles.

15

MERVYN SCHACHT

The Technique of Employing Doctor-Patient Transactions in Psychoanalysis

This article was stimulated by a recent paper of Dr. Hyman Fingert entitled "Comments on the Psychoanalytic Significance of the Fee."[1] Dr. Fingert focuses on the point that "the financial arrangements a patient makes for paying medical fees in psychoanalytic treatment usually reveal important facets of his character." He reviews the literature on the psychodynamics of money and its relation to the psychoanalytic fee, referring to the observations of Freud, Abraham, Fenichel, Jones, Lentino and others. He then summarizes two cases in order to illustrate the dynamics involved and to demonstrate how certain particular therapeutic procedures served to promote the emergence of the material, the mobilization of related effect, and the kind of insight that led to change and progress. In his cases, the patients did not want to pay their own fees, although they could afford to do so. They preferred, each according to his traits, to leave payment to their respective wealthy fathers. Dr. Fingert dealt with this directly and encouraged them to pay in cash from their own funds. As a result, analyzable material, previously unsubmitted, came into the open, and the treatment progress was facilitated significantly.

The present author has had several opportunities to observe how a real transaction between patient and doctor, such as that involving the fee, can be directly and effectively employed in furthering the treatment of the patient. In the cases described below, a fee situation

Reprinted with permission of the publisher from the *American Journal of Psychotherapy,* 1953, Vol. 7, 653-663.

1. Fingert, Hyman H.: *Bulletin of the Menninger Clinic,* Vol. 16, No. 3, May 1952, pp. 98-104.

was employed in such a manner as to elicit significant material and to promote insight that proved quite helpful to the patient.

Case Illustration #1

A 34-year-old, single woman entered psychoanalytic treatment complaining that she could not fall in love and marry although she wanted to do so. She functioned adequately in a responsible position and was earning a good salary. She enjoyed a busy social life, was liked and respected by all, and felt well adjusted. She emphasized that she had adequate sexual activity with good orgasms. She did not enter treatment with an initially recommended analyst because she felt she could not afford his fee. In turn, she was recommended to the present one who agreed to start treatment at a lowered fee.

The kind of resistance this patient was to manifest might have been anticipated from the initial interview. She acknowledged her inability to experience feelings of love and the fact that she required treatment for it; yet she felt well adjusted. She was a responsible person and serious about her intentions regarding treatment. She was strict in her values and therefore scrupulously honest in bringing up all the facts of her experiences for the analytic sessions. Yet, her mode of bringing up these experiences, her mode of viewing them and of viewing her role in them were always of such a nature as to undermine her own serious purposes and those of the analysis. She early introduced material lending to the interpretations that she was not able to express or advance her own desires in her relations with others. She was always doing favors and running errands. She over extended herself to obtain special discounts for her clients and felt guilty when requesting the smallest fees. She argued with no one and praised everyone. However, she could not see her activity in the light of this interpretation, and her mode of presenting the material made it hard for her to see it this way. Thus, she would tell of the resentment she felt at her roommate's excessive demands on her, and berate herself for this resentment. Careful examination verified that the roommate was morbidly dependent and that the patient was not refusing her demands. The patient emphasized her resentment, and the physician pointed toward an understanding of her inability to assert herself justly. Her response was in this vein, "Well, it's not that important. I can't take issue with every petty thing that comes up; I don't want to make it important. If I start asserting myself in these things I might go overboard and become a nasty person. Maybe my resentment indicates a hostile, selfish streak which has to come out in the analysis. I know another person would not be so unselfish but I'm afraid I might hurt my roommate, and I can't hurt anyone."

In brief then, the patient did inform the physician of her concern about her inability to assert herself, although she did it only indirectly and defended herself against the acknowledgment of such a disability. Also, she did respond to the physician's observation. She began to take just issue with her roommate. She curbed her inclination to do favors automatically and indiscriminately. She expressed more openly the facts that she did many a favor she did not really want to do, that people sometimes exploited this readiness on her part, that her friendships were based too largely on this single premise. With each such step she insisted that she was making unimportant issues important and substituting selfishness in the place of a concern for others. She also permitted the physician to see that her kindness had a definitely indiscriminate quality; that she could not, in the face of a choice, select a closer friend for a favor over a lesser acquaintance; that she complied with a person's request even when, in her judgment the asker wanted something that was not good for him. Her defense here was always, "How can I give my ideas and tell others what to do? How do I know I'm right?" She viewed herself as never having an opinion on most matters, as being unable to grasp the mechanism for formulating opinions. In gatherings she felt dull and superficial whereas others seemed "remarkably brilliant." At the same time she could not "understand" why others got "exercised" over various topics of discussion. Initially she said that she did not experience critical thoughts and feelings; later she said she could not express them because she did not "want to have them." These facts led to the interpretations: (a) That she was not devoid of feelings but rather employed devices to suppress them, (b) That she was disabled not only for fear of hurting others but for fear of any kind of participation, even at the expense of hurting others.

The patient did not acknowledge these insights verbally, but her behavior changed in accordance with them. As it did, she became increasingly anxious. She reported headaches and insomnia and consulted a general practitioner. She developed incapacitating fatigue and on a few occasions remained in bed all day, not going to work. Twice she lost her purse with sizable sums in it. These were unique experiences for this well organized person. They upset her and she insisted, "I can't let such things happen to me." The physician suggested that she was in an anxious state and encouraged her to examine her anxiety. She had previously emphasized that she did not know what anxiety felt like. She said now, "I don't feel anxious. I know I'm crying a lot lately, but I don't know why. I just seem to dissolve. Maybe that's what has to happen. By crying something is coming out and some kind of change is taking place in me."

In summation, the patient could not see the part that she played in what was taking place in her life, at the same time that she resisted seeing and resisted taking part. She often repeated, "I don't see how this treatment works or what is going on in it. I presume you could tell me everything but want me to go through all this. I know I'm getting something out of this but I can't say exactly what. I can say things more freely now; I don't do everything others ask and I feel freer for it. It's just that you gave me permission, and J. did too. It's wonderful–you both tell me that it's perfectly all right to say 'no.' "

J. was a man four years her senior with whom she established a relationship during this period. She had had a number of unrewarding relationships in the past. She had known J. for several years, had had some dates with him, always admired him and mentioned him as a prospect for marriage. He never indicated strong interest. The truth was that she had been unencouraging. More recently he initiated several dates. She was more responsive and they established a sexual relationship. Within a few months she complained that she was ready, for the first time, to have a truly close relationship but that J. put limits on it. The physician asked why she did not discuss this with him. She protested, "I can't make him do something he's not ready for; maybe it'll hurt him. I can't impose myself." Nonetheless, she did hesitantly voice her complaints and he responded quickly. He saw her daily and treated her seriously. He gave indications of an interest in marriage, suggesting that some personal problems were holding him up. The patient was thrown into maximum conflict. She had genuine feeling for this man and she was happy with the success of her initiative. But her anxiety prevented her from encouraging him further and she could not appreciate that she was anxious. She felt better than ever before in many ways, feeling herself especially to be a more definite person. Yet she reflected anxiety in somatic symptoms, in feeling grossly unworthy of her suitor, feeling torn apart and in spells of crying whenever he praised her.

In this period, she one day remarked that she felt guilty about the fee she was paying because she had friends in analysis paying higher fees. She has so remarked once or twice before but could not be encouraged to further exploration. This time the physician said, "As a matter of fact, I should like to discuss with you the possibility of an increase in fee." She responded, "There's nothing to discuss. If your fee is higher, I'll gladly pay it. I don't want to be paying you less than your regular fee; it's not fair." The physician expressed appreciation but emphasized that he was, in this instance, calling for a discussion of her thoughts and feelings on the subject. This discussion continued therafter, intermittently, for a period of six weeks. The patient introduced it in session after session. She stated frankly that the subject disturbed her. She could think of nothing to discuss regarding it, but she could not tolerate the fact that it remained an unsettled matter. She said, "This is a real issue between you and me; this is not analysis." She was anxious to get it settled as soon as possible. Headaches and insomnia increased.

For the first time in analysis she could see that she was experiencing anxiety and in what connection. She could see that she was anxious to pay an increase, not only on the basis of fairness but to close discussion of the matter. She managed, however, to pursue a discussion in the face of this anxiety. Initially, she could not validate her guilt feeling or specify what called for a fee increase. She could not specify what was valuable about the analysis; what she had learned about herself; what results such knowledge yielded, and in what way. As the discussion progressed, she came to see that she was incapable of specificity, not because the facts were missing or her mind limited, but because her mode of functioning was to remain as vague and unformulated about the facts as possible. Specificity made her uncomfortable. She was honest and perceptive enough to report guilt feeling regarding the fee, but when she said she was guilty she had completed her part. Either the subject would be dropped or the physician would decide about an increase. If he decided against it, he was depriving himself; if he decided for it, he was fulfilling his own requirements. For her part, she had no requirements in this regard at all. The physician in this instance, by requiring further exploration before agreeing to any decision, made it necessary for the patient to reach a clear picture of her own mode of behavior. He also obliged her to be quite specific before he lent agreement to her passive "unselfishness." It was only after she could provide appropriate indications for the change, and demonstrate that it was consistent both with the physician's and her own requirements (financial and other) that the physician acceded. When she finally instituted the increase, she did something perhaps for the first time knowing clearly why she did it, knowing its relationship to her own needs as well as to that of the other person, and knowing exactly how she felt about it.

This protracted piece of analytic work had healthy effects. The patient achieved insight regarding the particular quality and implications of her passive unselfishness. She wanted to be a selfless person, without personal goals and demands, always ready to do for others. She did, in fact, do many helpful things. But in denying personal demands, she could remain free of responsibility regarding the help she offered, and free of any significant involvement growing out of that help. She always expressed "willingness" to help; she never expressed "wanting" to help. She did not have to give thoughtful consideration as to exactly how constructive was the help she offered, and she could offer just as much help to one person as to another. No one person really mattered. She came to see how this approach left her isolated, and unable to protect herself; perpetuated feelings of unworthiness; kept her feeling guilty, prevented her from exercising independent judgment and from expressing feelings for another person. With this awareness, she became more goal directed, obtained better fees for her work and selected jobs that promised more personal satisfaction. She admitted that although she always considered money unimportant, she was most meticulous in organizing and going over her accounts each month. She recognized how her concern about money was denied in one area and verified in another. She went on to analyze her attitudes regarding money. She continued, in the face of anxiety which she could acknowledge, to work toward marriage, which did take place. Then she could acknowledge sexual difficulties with her husband, and contrary to her initial statement, sexual difficulties which antedated her relationship with her husband. She could then proceed to an analysis of them. She also became free to engage in constructive criticism or certain of her husband's behavior to which he responded positively, to their mutual satisfaction. She ultimately reached clarity as to what her analytic treatment and her improvement consisted of–viz. she was taking an increasingly active and determining part in what went on in her life.

Case Illustration # 2

A 27-year-old man entered psychoanalytic treatment for the first time complaining of recurring attacks of anxiety to the point of panic, associated with the thought and impulse to kill his wife. He had suffered from the same anxiety and obsession, directed toward others, from age fourteen and had always kept it a secret. He was raised on a farm and obliged by his father to work unduly long, hard hours, deprived of play and youthful friendships. A younger brother was always excused from chores, making the patient envious and revengeful. Also the brother often teased him, but being older and stronger the patient could not justly retaliate. In practice, he was on good terms with his brother and always considerate of him; but it was in regard to his brother that he first experienced the anxiety and the secret obsession. He left the farm when he was graduated from high school and the brother was never again the object of the obsession. He developed skill as an electronics technician but never held a job more than a few months. He felt painfully tied down, got panicky and quit. Also, any authority exerted over him was intolerable; he became anxious, experienced the impulse and quit. He was subject to paroxysms of loneliness which came over him suddenly, even during conversation, and he would remain miserable until he could think of something or do something pleasing to him. Sexual intercourse served in this way. He felt comforted by it and it was the one way he could appreciate a sensation of closeness with another person. It thus became a significant goal for him. He was proud when he could get a girl to participate, yet with success he became anxious and broke off. He was proud of his physique and strolled on the beach for all to admire him. He practiced weight lifting and body building exercises. At 21, he was inducted for army service but, after three weeks, became so panic stricken by the authority, discipline and close quarters with others that he required hospitalization and a medical discharge. He married at 26, after a courtship of six months. He became anxious on the honeymoon and experienced the thought and impulse to kill his wife. He was able to finish the honeymoon, set up home with his in-laws and get a job. After a few months on the job, his thought was that his wife was forcing him to stay on it and he felt an impulse to strangle her. This frightened him. He told his wife he was in a nervous state and she helped him get treatment. In the wife's eyes, the patient, although too reserved, was a considerate and an adequate husband.

In the initial interview the patient was soft spoken, unassertive and detached. His panic was not apparent although he described feelings of panic and confusion, and relief at the prospect of therapy. As treatment sessions progressed he never manifested overt discomfort. However, for the first three months he reported a succession of terrifying dreams in which he battled armies and hordes of ferocious beasts. For his productions, he gave detailed descriptions of his symptoms, relating them not to his feelings or activity but to the weather, time of the week, holidays and so forth. He appeared not to respond to the physician's attempt to have him relate them to his own life. He did not yield a clear picture of conflicts or personality problems. He rarely made reference to a previous session. He talked vaguely of the kind of person he thought himself to be. He would say, "I'm the kind of a guy who likes to be free. I couldn't take the Army because I can't be cooped up or disciplined. I don't like any bosses; I can't be tied down. I can do a favor if I volunteer it, not if it's asked. Things must be my way. I'm extremely meticulous; I can't drop a job unless it is perfect. I can't trust another person. I know I can rely on myself to be here each time but I can never rely on you; you can always decide to quit. I go by right and wrong a great deal. When I'm right I feel very secure; when I'm not right, I'm on shaky ground and can't say a thing. There are certain things about me I like and wouldn't want to change." With the physician, he was cooperative, even deferential. He rarely missed a session.

It became clear that this patient tried to establish his self-esteem in terms of grandiose and perfectionistic ideas and phantasies which he had developed. The ideas contained elements, however, which were potentially quite useful to him. He had a desire for good work performance, to do the right thing regarding other people, to be like others, to be mentally healthy, and to enjoy fruitful relationships. Early therapeutic activity was directed toward these elements and largely supportive. The physician focused attention on the symptoms as an expression of anxiety. He indicated that the patient's distaste for being tied down and for authority were really anxiety about these things; that he was anxious about authority, in spite of good work, because of his own needs for perfection; that he wanted to be free of bonds to be an object of universal admiration. He indicated, for the patient, what might be productive as contrasted with what tended to be self-defeating about these reactions and modes of behavior. He related his dreams to the analysis.

The patient remained on his job, got successive raises and was ultimately elevated to foreman in charge of 40 employees. His terrifying dreams disappeared. He left his in-laws to take an apartment of his own, although initially anxious over this prospect. His wife gave birth in a planned pregnancy, and he enjoyed the child, although at first he had feared having one. He never volunteered any remarks about the treatment, however, or his progress in it. At one time, when asked, he said that he felt less in awe of other people, less inferior and friendlier. He kept to himself less and had a feeling of real ability. He had definitely matured, and others had noticed the difference in him. However, he was not clear about these changes and could not be gotten to elaborate on them. Repeated attempts by the physician to encourage a discussion of what the patient was experiencing in his analysis were unsuccessful. In fact, as he progressed the patient became vaguer and more repetitious in delineating symptoms and in describing what he thought he was like. And the more he improved, the greater became the discrepancy between the way he was living and his ideas about himself. The physician submitted this for exploration. The patient replied that he did not put emphasis on the improvements he described. His thoughts were on his symptoms. He figured he would have worked out his personality problems without treatment if he had not had symptoms. He admitted, when asked what he had lately been experiencing, occasional feelings of anger and disappointment regarding the physician which he left unmentioned. He said he maintained the physician as an unreal person in his own thinking to make it possible for him to trust and confide; personal reactions he blotted out of mind.

The physician observed: (a) That the patient maintained certain illusions for himself, and (b) that he was a secretive person who was discussing one set of facts in analysis and keeping another set to himself. The patient acknowledged these observations but could examine them only abortively.

The patient was in treatment on a reduced fee because he had been in financial straits at the onset. One day, after a year of analysis, he said, "This treatment is great stuff. My boss gave me another raise. Now, I'm earning twice as much as when I started." He was sure the treatment was a responsible factor but he could not elaborate on the connection and soon dropped the subject. Shortly thereafter the physician said, "I would like to discuss with you the possibility of an increase in fee." The patient was silent for some minutes, then, in a quiet voice said, "I'm very angry. I feel trapped. No way out. I need the treatment and must depend on you. Things are pretty tight, with the baby and the apartment. I couldn't tell my wife, she's complaining about the expense already. I'll have to cut out lunches, not use my allowance, figure out other ways to accumulate the money." This was the only discussion he could offer. After the hour he asked, "Do you want me to start the increase now?" The physician repeated that it was a discussion he was calling for. The patient was visibly relieved. He did not reintroduce it for further discussion. He returned to the old themes. He again remarked that he could trust no one and had to see to everything himself. The physician said, "This is doubtful. You were ready to pay an increase last week without questioning why it should be, or how much. If it depended on you or if your physician were untrustworthy, you would be paying it already. You appear to *think* of yourself as behaving in a certain way, but your actual behavior can be different." In the sessions immediately following, the physician had repeated opportunities to employ the patient's response in the fee discussion in the manner of the example above. The patient would talk vaguely of his independence, of his inclination to cooperate only when he volunteered it, of his firmness when he felt he was right, and so forth. The physician would then recall the patient's actual response to the fee discussion, and delineate the discrepancy between the thought and the act. In a short time the patient began to appreciate the significance of this and to contribute illustrations of his own that corroborated and extended this insight. He volunteered that when reality contradicted his illusions, he did what was right or realistic, and he blocked out of mind any consideration of the contradiction. He did not like to be bossed, but whenever the boss requested him to stay overtime, he never objected. He did not like to take assistance from another person on the job, but he never failed to accept it when advisable. When his child was born he was close to panic momentarily in contemplating the burdens and responsibilities involved. He then blocked it out of mind and it returned in the form of an apparently unexplainable impulse directed at the child. When he realized this, he could also realize that he was handling this responsibility quite well and did not require escapist illusions as a source of self esteem. He volunteered that he had always tried to impress his wife that he had been a ladies' man before marriage but that this was untrue. He added other inaccurate impressions he had tried to make on his wife, the physician and others. He was able to tell the physician on the spot, after a given interpretation, that he felt the impulse toward him. This was a unique experience in confiding for this patient and it was followed by a fruitful exploration of his feelings regarding the physician and the analysis. He saw that he was secretly taking improvement from analysis on the one hand and retaining his illusions on the other. Since the facts belied the illusions, they only served to perpetuate his anxiety and obsessions. Following these insights, there evolved a change in the quality of the patient's participation in therapy. He became more candid in acknowledging and discussing his various feelings, modes of thought and conflicts. He developed interest in the continuity of the analysis and in the concrete role it was playing in his life. Discussion of symptoms fell off and the symptoms themselves abated. Simultaneously he reintroduced the question of the fee. He was able to describe those of his thoughts and feelings that came into play, as this subject was discussed. His retentiveness regarding money and its relationship to other aspects of his personality was brought out. He could then proceed to a more realistic discussion of all the factors involved relative to a raise in fee. This time he brought out a financial problem he was facing, heretofore unknown to the analyst. A fee raise was agreed upon but it was postponed until a specific time in the future when his financial problem would be solved. This provided the patient with further evidence of the possibilities that lay in being confidential and dealing cooperatively with another person, as against his own inclinations to secretiveness and illusory independence.

Conclusion

Psychoanalytic technique requires that real transactions between patient and physician be kept at a minimum. However, the transactions that are necessary, such as those involving the payment of fees, do not by their nature interfere with the therapeutic process. On the contrary, they are ingredient and contributory parts of the treatment and can serve as valuable sources of exploration and insight. In this author's experience, there have been instances wherein adhering exclusively to the technique of interpreting only the patient's spontaneously offered free associations has failed to overcome sustained resistance. In at least some of these, the resistance appears to have been related to some concrete doctor-patient situation that had not yet been adequately explored. When, as in the cases described in this paper, it was possible to invoke an examination of that concrete situation, insight emerged, resistance was overcome and progress once again ensued.

The analytic exploration of doctor-patient transactions, fee or any other, has proved repeatedly to be a most useful technique. Perhaps the fact that there are so few of them, lends them so well to this use. They provide excellent examples for reality testing; the physician has a first hand opportunity to know the situation that is being analyzed. They serve to bring home to the patient that the analysis is not an academic, but a real and serious procedure. They permit the patient to feel much more on a par with the physician. Too often a patient feels inferior to the physician because he is riddled with questionable motivations while his analyst, in defining these very motivations for him, seems quite free of material motivations and thereby perfect. Exploration of real transactions permits the patient to realize that the physician has requirements and motivations of his own; and that these can nonetheless be consistent with the welfare of the patient. The author has seen patients' self esteem elevated through such exploration. The patient comes to see more clearly the contributions that he has been making toward a successful result.

Dr. Fingert used a method of direction with his patients. The present author used a somewhat different technique, but an extension of the same principle. He held up the completion of the actual transaction to encourage an analytic exploration of it and the patient's unconscious motivations connected with it. The withholding served to make exploration and insight a virtual consequence. It had the advantage, perhaps, that when the transaction was finally effected, the patient acted neither blindly nor on authority, but out of full awareness—the ultimate desideratum of psychoanalysis. It had the advantage, too, that it promoted insight not only into the psychodynamics of money, but into other conflictual and defensive patterns of the patient.

16

GREGORY ZILBOORG

Emotional Engagement of Patient and Analyst

Following an oft-repeated analogy, one may say that the relationship between analysand and psychoanalyst during treatment is similar to the one between the surgeon and his patient: The field of operation must be and remain aseptic throughout the therapeutic procedure. However, even under the strictest control of conditions in the operating room, foolproof asepsis cannot be achieved; moreover, even if a contamination of one kind or another happens to fail to affect the successful outcome of a given operation, other factors which have nothing to do with infectious agents may directly affect the patient who is under the knife of the surgeon—the person of the surgeon, for instance. If he be anxious and tense or otherwise inclined to be "subjective," or lacking in gentleness, he may pull the tissues a bit too hard, press the organs a bit too "roughly," be too hurried when prudence would require deliberate slowness, or be too unhurried when the condition of the patient seemed to require an acceleration of pace. All these things are not merely a matter of technique or skill; they are often, if not preeminently, a matter of the personality of the surgeon, of his psychological makeup.

In other words, even in surgery the psychological condition of those who work in the operating room seems to be of great importance—this in the presence of even the most accomplished skill and the most complete asepsis. In psychoanalytic work (and this is true nowadays of any psychotherapeutic procedure) the "personal equa-

Reprinted from Jules Masseman (ed.), *Science and Psychoanalysis* (New York, Grune & Stratton, 1960) Vol. 3, 260-270.

tions" of the psychoanalyst, and these alone, are the factors responsible for the proper calm, poise and so-called "objective" handling of the issues involved, without which considerable failures or unforeseen and undesirable aftereffects will result.

We must remember that, platitudinous as all this may sound now, psychoanalysis was originally not at all aware of the importance of the personality of the analyst or his state of mind at any given moment during the psychoanalytic treatment. Such terms as "the psychoanalytic situation" were introduced much later, and the very phenomenon of transference was discussed for many years with apparent detachment until years of experience forced the psychoanalyst to recognize or, shall we say, to admit the existence of countertransference. Freud from the outset cultivated his psychoanalytic approach in accordance with the pattern of the biologically oriented medical man. A patient was a patient and could and must therefore be looked upon with almost frigid objectivity, somewhat in the manner of the pathologist performing an autopsy. But a corpse is a corpse—not a living person—and the pathologist can proceed with his work without any fear of death, or without any compassion for the one who suffered and died and was brought to the dissecting table.

It is hardly necessary to recapitulate the history of the development of insight into the psychoanalyst's relationship to his psychoanalytic work. Suffice it to say that throughout this history there seemed to be little doubt in the best psychoanalytic minds that the lofty objectivity of Nirvana could be achieved, and by way of the very psychoanalytic technique which had theretofore appeared insufficient because the psychoanalyst was not sufficiently trained, not sufficiently analyzed, not free of his own neurosis, etc. True, Freud, whose intuition was always ahead of that of his best disciples, already toward the end of the third decade of our century thought it desirable that psychoanalysts themselves undergo a sort of psychoanalytic checkup every five years or so. But even with this insight into the frailty of the psychoanalyst's psychological makeup, the general, even though unspoken, attitude seems to have been that the patient was an object of investigation—psychologically unstable, emotionally fickle or hard-boiled and stubborn, in constant need of correction, of being changed or modified—and that the psychoanalyst, after his own analysis had been finished, was fit to do the job, provided he every now and then brushed up on the technique in order to keep in trim.

The history of psychoanalysis during the last fifteen or twenty years, particularly in America, is replete with telling illustrations of the vicissitudes of the difficulties which psychoanalysts suffer at the hands of their patients, and patients at the hands of their psychoanalysts. These illustrations are not always presented as actual cases. As with so many other things in the psychoanalytic movement, the difficulties are expressed in the form of disagreement as to theory, or in the form of "splits," of all sorts of "schismatic" structures under the flag of abandoning the "orthodoxy" whose positive dogma is not always clear. Some have rejected transference–concept, phenomena, et al.; some would reject the Oedipus complex; others would drive the term anxiety to its extreme existential depth so as to abondon Freud's initial and ultimate concept of anxiety, which at the beginning at least was abstract rather than phenomenologic. The concomitant of all these denials and rejections was a certain bitterness; although on many occasions this bitterness remained hidden under the toga of psychoanalytic objectivity, it was always harsh.

Granted that the patient and his troubles come first; granted that the psychoanalyst's training is very important; granted all this, there is left the hidden and the unaccountable mass of the psychoanalyst's character traits. I have in mind the constants, "the unanalyzable" elements of the psychoanalyst's personality which are not neurotic, so to speak, and which are and always will be determinants in the development and the resolution of the psychoanalytic situation.

Heretofore, what seems to have been considered decisive and most dangerous was the psychoanalyst's possible sexual involvement with his patient: The inability of the psychoanalyst to stand the pressure of the countertransference in the sexual field, with a corresponding acting out, in the literal sense of that countertransference. Some flagrant and tragic cases of this kind became known to the public, and some even became a matter of historical annotation. Jones reported in considerable detail the Frink case, for instance. Freud's attitude in this respect was interesting: He loved Frink; he considered him a most gifted man, particularly in psychoanalysis; Frink's falling in love with one of his patients, his divorce and his ultimate psychosis were all treated by Freud with utmost tolerance at the time. All Frink's difficulties did not seem to Freud to disqualify the good psychoanalyst that he saw in him. One wonders whether the superstitious prejudice of the general public endowing every analyst with the capacity of establishing a liaison with every woman patient, did not stem from the open tolerance toward cases like Frink's at the turn of the century. With the years, Freud's attitude appears to have undergone considerable change, as testified by the emphatic letter of warning Freud wrote to Ferenczi when the full import of Ferenczi's innovations in the technique of psychoanalysis became clear to him.

It is natural, of course, that the sexual aspects of the countertransference should have come first (albeit a bit late) to the attention of clinical psychoanalysts. But, if we abandon for a moment the narrow meaning of countertransference and turn our attention to some general characteristics of the relationship between psychoanalyst and patient, some things will come to light which have been only vaguely noted, if at all, by psychoanalysts during the past half century.

Take, for instance, the psychoanalyst who is of a scholarly bent of mind, a great reader, a man of considerable scientific curiosity. For all intents and purposes let us consider him a normal, "nonneurotic" person. He is a wonderful example of what appears to be a perfectly sublimated voyeurism, which makes him a keen, perspicacious psychoanalyst. His listening to patients is irreproachable. As a matter of fact his listening to patients is to him *the* sublimation of his voyeurism. Consequently, he feels no urge to say much, no need to give many interpretations, no need to become active. As long as his curiosity (the unconscious voyeurism) is being gratified, he can remain the very ideal of psychoanalytic passivity and orthodoxy. On the other hand, voyeur that he is, he cares comparatively little about what really happens to his patients. In other words, his objectivity is really indifference. Voyeurism is not a strictly object-libidinous orientation. Hence, once his sagacious mind "understands" the patient, i.e., once his voyeurism is satisfied, there is little of "the therapeutic intent" that would drive him along. A "good" psychoanalytic diagnosis suffices; it satisfies his interest, his wish to "look in." It is obvious that the relationships between such an analyst and his patients are good, inoffensive, undisturbed, unmarred by any dramatic difficulties. Some of those patients will get well, some will not, but the psychological ties between such a therapist and his patients are bound to remain tenuous, as are the ties between those patients and their fellow men.

It is of no importance now to assess the values of such relationships, particularly the therapeutic values. It is doubtful whether at the present state of our knowledge and the great diversity of theoretical approaches it would be possible to say with any degree of certainty which particular attitude in which person will bring about which therapeutic result. We may recall in the connection the words of Kretschmer some thirty years ago about the recovery of schizophrenics, that he had no objection whatsoever to the patient's keeping to himself a few *private* hallucinations and delusions, provided he maintained his social recovery.

One need not be a therapeutic perfectionist to find oneself objecting to Kretschmer's rather simplified sociologic appraisal of mental health. On the other hand, one can hardly be accused of therapeutic nihilism if one bears in mind that the person of the psychoanalyst has a profound, unalterable and ineffaceable bearing on the form and manner of the given patient's therapeutic success. Call it unconscious identification with the therapist, call it unconscious imposition of the therapist's attitude on the patient, call it the interaction (unconscious) between the two psychologies the fact remains that the therapist is never able fully to attain that lofty Olympian objectivity which borders on haughty pedestrian indifference. If such objectivity-indifference could be achieved, he would have to devise some potent methods to avoid it, for it would lead to personal stagnation and to therapeutic sterility.

We thus are inevitable led to the conclusion that that which for want of another term we would call the personal equation of the therapist is, and actually must be, the totality of the therapist's affective propensities or biases which in some way become integrated with his intuitive keenness and the sum total of his sense of values, or morality if you wish. It is this integrated complexity that is charged with a great deal of affect even in the "coolest" and most poised therapists, and it is this affective charge, so intimately personal and unconscious, that embodies both the therapeutic intent and the sense of conviction with which the therapeutic process is being carried out. It is this intimately personal element of the therapist which is responsible for all the good and all the bad which can be found in psychotherapy in general and in psychoanalysis in particular. And it is this complex component of the therapist which is responsible not only for the multiple divisions and subdivisions in the history of psychoanalysis, but also for the ill-concealed sense of property so many therapists show in the business of recruiting collaborators; it is this same component that produces that form of assent which to so-called outsiders, or dissidents, appears but a blind passivity. For the sake of truth in general and candor and scientific probity in particular, it is incumbent upon us to admit that many of the fervid disciples of so many not less fervid leaders are born in an atmosphere of possessiveness and carried on the illusory wings of some sort of power which is only euphemistically called leadership.

There is little doubt in my mind that the above description corresponds to the psychological truth, although there is also little doubt in my mind that there is neither dishonesty nor perversity in the manifestation to which I have tried to allude. At worst we might call it all the general weakness of man seen even in psychoanalysis; at best it is an expression of fervor in which it is at times difficult to differentiate the woof of the missionary from the warp of the propagandist, both wearing respectfully and respectably the cloak of scientific thought. A few years ago Jules Masserman did an excellent job of evoking from the past the old picture of the travails of the phrenologic movement and reminding us of some of the corresponding features of present-day psychoanalysis. I would like on this occasion to express my assent to Masserman's skillful historical excursion and would wish here to make but one change: I would use the term "psychoanalyses"—in the plural.

Bearing in mind the above psychological limitations (and they are serious ones) on the objectivity of the therapist in relation to his patient, it will not be difficult for us to conclude that the psychological engagement between patient and therapist is of an affective, moral nature; it is not of necessity a positive relationship, and it carries within itself dangers which do not necessarily lie in the overflow of positive feelings alone, from the so-called countertransference in the narrow sense of the word. At times danger comes to an even greater extent from the negative feelings, for after all positive feelings can be admitted into consciousness more readily when they may assume in our eyes a form of sympathy, or compassion, or that which we call "understanding." Moreover, we do seem even consciously inclined to cultivate that type of understanding between analyst and patient. A few purely private fantasies beyond the borders of this understanding might even be permitted to appear to our mind, provided they remain private.

It is different and more difficult when we come to hostility. Barring exceptional cases in which hostility seems unavoidable and justified, it is difficult if not impossible to have our hostility toward a patient appear to us in the cloak of objectivity. A conservative psychoanalyst might find it difficult to keep his composure if he attempts to analyze a Communist; a Jewish psychoanalyst would find it impossible to hold his hatred in check if he were to discover that his patient served at one time as an assistant in a Nazi mass crematorium. Under "normal" circumstances hostility toward a patient can be kept in check only if repressed into the unconscious. Thus it may appear on the surface as a mild depressive complaint that there is a very difficult patient at hand, it may appear in the form of a rather intensive interpretation of the patient's narcissism, but almost never as true hostility. This hostility being repressed might have a cumulative effect; years later it might even appear in the form of a legal or quasi-legal prosecution of a former patient. Rare as such cases are, they are very instructive; they demonstrate how brittle yet how intense is a relationship based on unconscious hostility. Under no other circumstances do human relationships suffer to such an extent. Franz Alexander many years ago in Berlin aptly spoke of this joining in battle of hostilities which is involved in psychoanalysis as *die Narzissmen reiben sich*—the reciprocal friction between (or among) narcissisms.

It would require a great deal of time and space to enumerate all or even most of the variations of human frailties which put pitfalls in the path of our therapeutic efforts. It would seem that under the heading of Eros and Hate most of the difficulties of psychoanalytic therapy would find their proper place. It is obvious that this is as it always has been, in human life and in the relationships between human beings. There is a difference, however: In general human relationships, the sociologic and ethical factors become inevitably involved and these more or less normalize, or at any rate stabilize for certain periods of time, the life and the living of human society. However, in the human relationship called the psychoanalytic situation, or the interrelationship between patient and therapist, the sociologic and ethical pressures seem to be attenuated in their normative sense and put at the disposal of the field of affective life and that measure of cool reason which the psychoanalyst presumably always possesses and the patient potentially has. In other words, the field of operation is from the outset contaminated with affective charges, and its being thus contaminated becomes the very condition under which the psychotherapeutic procedure must progress almost to its very end.

All this puts an unusual burden on the moral stability of the therapist. It would seem that the phenomenologic, or existential (they are not exactly the same, of course), school of psychoanalysis was born out of the need to make this burden easier. The so-called existential analysis centers its attention on the patient and the outside world, two complexities of interaction, and it is the neurosis that is considered the masterful perverter of the world. The existential psychotherapist is therefore from the very beginning a self-confessed outsider too, and as such he may find that he might be less involved personally in the therapeutic process. But I, for one, doubt whether he can succeed in escaping the pitfalls of which I have spoken.

In all this discussion I have deliberately omitted a consideration of the great variety of pitfalls which patients themselves put in the way of the psychoanalyst. Their characterologic variety is great; their name is legion. They run the whole gamut from mute inaccessibility to deliberate seductiveness, from pious self righteousness to confessions of murders actually committed but heretofore undiscovered. The many fascinating and revolting varieties of pitfalls would not affect the general considerations brought forward here and the few conclusions to be offered. All varieties of this sort may be grouped under the heading: The troubles which patients choose to confide to the psychoanalyst and the burden of irreproachable, unwavering discretion which they put on the analyst.

It might occur to some that it is wrong to consider the need for discretion a severe, or any kind of, burden. At first glance this thought appears quite correct; discretion in medical, and particularly in medico-psychological, work is a moral attribute which should not be difficult to acquire by a professional man and ought not to be hard to keep. Our patients do trust us and, despite their hesitations, anxieties and suspicions, they acquire—or generate—full confidence in us. They thus encourage us, because their faith in us enhances within us the obligation and the need to be discreet. This aspect of the relationship between psychoanalysts and their patients is frequently overlooked by the general public and even by a large section of the medical profession, who do not understand that the confidence placed in analysts by patients awakens in analysts the moral forces which demand that they be discreet and live up to the best levels of that confidence.

But as far as I know, analysts have viewed this phenomenon only from the standpoint of what it does to (how harmful it is for) the patient's analysis. What it does to the psychoanalyst appears to be a totally neglected question. Patients seem to be privileged to say whatever occurs to them to whomever happens to strike their fancy, and in whatever manner they happen to choose. If patients choose to speak, to boast of or to malign their analyst, the analyst learns about it sooner or later. It would not do at all to insist that the well trained and well analyzed psychoanalyst remain totally objective in such matters; it would not do to dispose of the matter by merely assuming that good professional training and a perfect training analysis make the analyst impervious to good public opinion and insensitive to bad public opinion. Such imperviousness would be a mark of an autistic character which any analyst can ill afford to possess, and such insensitiveness would mark the analyst as an even more autistic person than is good for everyday living, let alone everyday work with patients' emotions and minds.

It would seem that gradually but surely I have reached an impasse. The argument, it will have been noticed by now, was all in favor of bringing out the difficulties which psychoanalysts find in their work. What is worse, I seem to have argued that the psychoanalyst's reactions to the various reactions of his patients were somehow inevitable. Heretofore such reactions were considered "weaknesses" to be eliminated by the training analysis. In this consideration we were and are supported by a kind of silent belief in the therapeutic omnipotence of psychoanalysis.

But this is an omnipotence in which Freud himself did not believe. As is known, Freud was often skeptical of the therapeutic value of psychoanalysis. One wonders whether this skepticism is not even more justified in so-called normal cases—and people who choose to go into a training analysis may hardly be considered less than the usual, run-of-the-mill normal people, whatever their intellectual endowment.

We may not refuse to admit that patients represent a particular psychological burden to the analyst, and that the analyst must carry this burden with all its implications of subjectivity. I have in mind the burdens in everyday cases, not only in such exceptional situations as overlooking or otherwise failing to prevent the possible suicide of a patient. In such situations it is easy to see that the psychoanalyst's feelings toward the patient would naturally be a mixture of compassion and hositility; of course he would be sorry that the person under his care had killed himself: He would be sorry for the person who is dead and for himself, who under the circumstances becomes exposed to public opinion as a serious failure. I would make bold to say that the fear of a tragic outcome such as suicide, and the consequent admixture of hostility, may serve to repress the psychoanalyst's feeling and feed him "from within" with a kind of "affective therapeutic optimism," which might in great part be responsible for his blurred clinical vision and consequent sense of guilt. Such complex emotional constellations are not easy to decipher in a training analysis. They are more difficult to lay bare after such an analysis.

So much more difficult a complexity of affects with regard to the patient is the analyst subjected to in a number of other situations in which the patient is an active "spiller," so to speak. The indiscretions of the patients with regard to the psychoanalyst do not release the analyst from his obligation not to talk about the patient. In a case of suspected suicide, the analyst may and should feel free to break the seal of privileged communications and therefore of strict discretion and warn the next of kin or whomever he deems wise of the possible danger. In such a case the analyst would make an attempt to share his responsibilities with someone else; this produces an important condition of psychological alleviation for the analyst; his anxieties and his hostilities of the moment become attenuated.

The situation is entirely different when the patient chooses to "spill" and the analyst is or justifiably feels he is maligned, and there is actually no relief forthcoming. It is doubtful whether the analyst may under such circumstances drop his attitude of discretion. Moreover, he probably would not be able to reach the multiple ears of gossip and slander, even if he thought he might permit himself "to talk." Under such circumstances neither self-analysis, nor "more analysis," nor any other purely scientfic psychological procedure will prove of much avail.

It is evident that the moral fiber of the analyst is under greater stress than that of any other medical specialist. This is so much more true because the analyst's work has a more than serious effect on human relations; the effect is direct and potent and yet almost entirely elusive. The effect of the psychoanalyst's personality on the patient and the effect of psychoanalysis on the patient are conglomerated with many external circumstances, social and individual and not lending themselves to the understanding of even the most sagacious sociologist or psychologist.

In other words, we are dealing here with imponderables of the highest potency, one of the major components of which is the psychoanalyst who is, strictly speaking, left to himself, immersed in a mixture of obligations and emotions from discretion to hatred, from extreme personalism to most abstract culturalism—that is to say, from narrowest narcissism to highly socialized self consciousness, from psychological formalism to free-flowing, ethical intuitivism. The analyst, therefore, pending some great and miraculous discovery, has not only to fall back on his conscience, but to lean on it constantly and lean on it heavily, yet without pious moralism and self-righteous haughtiness in relation to his patients. A so-called good, or healthy (whatever it may mean) superego will hardly suffice, since the superego is not of ethical but mostly of punitive, hostile origin. I happen to belong to those who with Charles Odier would differentiate superego from conscience, and for this reason alone would not consider the superego by itself sufficient to help us in these our difficulties, unless it be a special, professional superego, tailored and fashioned in accordance with the needs of the psychoanalytic profession.

Since superegos cannot be made to order, nor conscience be a purely personal matter, it seems necessary for us to seek the solution of the problems before us not so much in purely scientific categories, but in the perennial absolutes which are found in morality and in the natural law in general. Unfortunately science as such has not yet found a way to make a permanent peace with the natural law. We shall remain hopeful that some day it will.

17

HANNA COLM

The Therapeutic Encounter

Part I

In recent years many different approaches to psychotherapy have developed from that prescribed by Freud. In broad lines Freud's view of the therapeutic relationship was: the patient revealing slowly to himself and to the analyst the buried feelings and impulses, which–pushed under–could not allow him to feel at one with himself. The analyst was merely a screen on which the patient projected his feelings–tender and hostile ones. The analyst himself stayed uninvolved and "accepting."

It was quite a revolutionary step forward in this country when Sullivan demanded "participant observation" from the analyst, and when later on, in carrying out this suggestion, the analyst discovered that he himself had at times countertransference reactions–reactions which originated in his own past. There followed a decade in which analysts tried to become aware of this countertransference and to "work it out," which really meant "work it away."

In recent years this developement moved in a different direction stimulated by existential philosophers, most of whom were not analysts but knew about the human being and the human condition. However, what we call existential psychotherapy developed not merely because certain philosophers influenced the thinking of analysts: it resulted from an experience of frustration both on the side of the patient and the analyst.

Patients began to object to the inhumanness and artificiality of

Reprinted with permission of the publisher from the *Review of Existential Psychology and Psychiatry*, Vol. V, 1965, 137-159.

this authoritatively, intellectually perceived prescription of the analyst who stayed uninvolved, not feeling, but pretended in a rather controlled way always to accept. Yet the uninvolved therapist was supposed to symbolize the lack of authoritative guidance or influence. To an increasing number of patients, it did not make sense that the trouble into which he had gotten through frustration should be cured by more frustration—by lack of response, lack of reaction, and by an acceptance which he could not feel to be genuine because it was a method merely learned by the analyst. How could such a controlled and prescribed therapeutic relationship heal the patient who may already suffer from lack of trust in genuine relationship to people?

Analysts also experienced that the attempt to control their counter-transference merely kept it out of sight. They also became aware that they really could not genuinely accept all and everything, that the Freudian demand "the analyst has to be in an attitude of full acceptance" made a robot rather than a healer of him.

Encouraged by Buber, Tillich, Heidegger, Binswanger, and Boss, among others, a number of European and American analysts dared to accept the fact that a genuine mutual relationship developed in the process of healing. They say that in a genuine partnership an understanding of the patient's difficulties could develop in a more spontaneous and honest, and therefore more helpful way.

The analyst's humanness is experienced by the patient in the treatment and plays a major part in restoring his feeling of integrity and trust. It gives the patient a chance to overcome his feeling of worthlessness which may have been acquired from childhood images of perfection and omnipotence.

Freud's intuition about, and his study of, human defenses still proved as valid as ever, yet Freud's approach to the patient was essentially changed—from "technique" to "interaction" and "encounter." No longer have we the contrast to the "patient," who does not know how to live, versus the "doctor," who is beyond all problems; but in treatment two human beings meet who struggle to accept the manifold human predicaments in which they both got entangled while trying to find a way out to the patient's difficulties. This changed approach became one of the expressions of existential thinking in the field of psychotherapy.

Substituting the genuine "encounter" for the analytical "technique" may be regarded as an ideal of existential therapy but is by no means achieved with each individual patient or in each individual hour. There are patients and hours in which also the existential therapist will use utmost restraint—it is perhaps the greatest difficulty in existential analysis to know when the patient is ready to be exposed to what may sometimes be the shock of genuine encounter.

What is involved in this therapeutic existential encounter for the patient and the therapist? The patient who has made up his mind to seek help from a therapist thereby alone proves a certain courage. It is the courage to face oneself and the willingness to have another person discover with him his real being of which he is only vaguely aware. This courage and willingness to run a risk gives the opening for the possibility of an encounter.

On the side of the therapist the initial difficulty might be even greater. For him the patient is initially "a case." He may have first a positive, negative, or indifferent feeling towards him. Perhaps he needs some "technique" which every therapist may develop in his own way for finding an access to the patient to prepare the ground on his side for an encounter. One such "technique" which I found fruitful is to listen and try to observe the patient's behavior and his symptoms, forgetting preconceived diagnostic patterns which so often lead us to overlook or overstress factors or see the patient in terms of a general pattern rather than how he *is*.

Secondly, while I listen—and this is very helpful to me—I try to look at his disturbed behavior not as "pathology," but in terms of what this behavior and what his symptoms possibly express in terms of their meaning to his whole living. What is it he tries to tell me? Often "neurotic behavior and symptoms" express as much as possible the degree to which a patient can live *with integrity* in an adverse family or cultural situation. I look not for his pathology but for his integrity.

This approach helps me to find thwarted yet basically positive angles in his behavior; it helps me to understand rebellious behavior as reaction to dependency on, and conformance with, a person who was experienced as an authority in childhood. This approach helps me often to overcome my own obstacles to open up for entering into the struggle with the patient's neurotic solutions.

In the process of this search for the patient's integrity, I observe as I do during the whole period of therapy what genuine reactions his behavior causes in *me*. It might well be the same adverse reaction which he often experiences from others, without being aware that he causes these reactions himself, at least partially. From sharing my personal reaction with him we can see more clearly the variety of reactions his behavior may bring about in others. My reaction and my willingness to reveal my reactions opens him up to a greater willingness to evaluate and communicate his own feelings.

Trying to see what is in *the patient* corresponds to trying to observe what is in terms of reaction in me. I use it as a starting point towards experiencing him and me in interaction, in a back and forth process of questioning both of us. In this process we both must be open to correct our experience of each other where it belongs to our past and is not a genuine reaction to the other person. This is the process which gradually heals, most of all the patient, but also the therapist, from leftover childhood ideals of perfection and the resulting disappointment about oneself, others, and life in general.

Healing does not result merely from greater *knowledge* of oneself but from *experiencing* oneself (as one *is*) in relation to another person and in the struggle towards mutual acceptance in spite of the humanness one finds in oneself and in one's partner. I am not afraid of letting counter-transferences enter into my reactions. I feel they are helpful if shared (1) in clarifying the reality of the interaction, and (2) in helping the patient and myself not to forget that counter-transferences–transferences from the past–belong to the human equipment. They can be of positive value–an immediate liking of a person, or they can be of an initial disturbance to a relationship and then offer an opportunity to be worked on.

These and similar techniques, useful as they are, should however only be regarded as bridges for crossing the initial gulf between the doctor and the patient.

Once a certain rapport has been established the therapist can go ahead of his patient in daring to be himself. He should be open for a genuine encounter in feeling, be it affection, or irritation, or even temporary hate, or the thousands of feelings that each patient will provoke in his therapist and the therapist in the patient.

At the right time the therapist will dare to show the patient that he too is only a human being who has his reactions, positive and negative, which the patient must learn to accept or refuse. Thus the patient, in the encounter with the therapist, must again become a full person and will gradually gain trust in his own judgement not only in his dealings with the therapist, but also in dealing with his own life situations.

Only an encounter–alive as this–will help the patient experience and accept the manifold positive and negative feelings in dealing with his family, colleagues, and so on.

The therapist offers himself to experience the patient's troubled way of living, but it would become a condescending, one-sided experience if he would not also want his patient to share his own reactions. Gradually the therapist can help the patient to recognize that the negative reactions he provokes in the therapist are similar to reactions he provokes in daily living and which may contribute to his frustrations. Very often the patient will show in the encounter with the therapist that unconsciously he tries to destroy genuine basic affection in fear of closeness. This again may lead him to recognize and instigate an attitude which may cause him difficulties in daily living.

In this process, patient and therapist will share their reactions to each other with an openness that "politeness" usually does not permit in our culture.

These reactions which patient and therapist must share consist to a large extent of expressions of hostility and distrust, but sometimes also of affection and tenderness. There will be long periods of indifference, where the therapist does not find that the time is ripe for an open expression and the patient is not ready on his side. Yet this openness is eventually necessary for the process of healing. Without it, the patient would not become aware of what his behavior and his symptoms provoke in others and where others might be hurt.

Sometimes the patient's behavioral problems become apparent in his relation to the therapist and also in accidental occurrences with other patients in the waiting room. In many cases in which husband-and-wife problems are involved it is highly useful to permit a three-cornered encounter to develop. In group therapy the interactions among various people are given their greatest chance for bringing out the problem in an actual life situation. I found it even useful sometimes to have my dog in the room, especially with children.

In the back and forth of the discussion of the patient's and therapist's reaction, both patient and therapist slowly get a glimpse of what the inner meaning of the patient's behavior and symptoms is. This does not mean that the patient learns that his behavior and symptoms are provocative and therefore he will be prudent enough to change his way of life. Rather, in a deeper way, he learns to recognize that his behavior and symptoms are a distorted outgrowth of what may be his basic integrity. What he initially may have grasped intellectually, eventually—in the ideal case—will through this process penetrate his person and contribute to his healing.

This result can only be achieved if the therapist reveals himself in this encounter to the patient not as authoritative, but in a joint undertaking as a partner who may possibly be mistaken. The therapist will show over and over that he is human himself and not beyond conflicts and failures.

The therapeutic encounter is centered around the patient's difficulties in living, but the therapist necessarily will be drawn into the process through his positive contributions, his interpretations, his impressions, his intuition, as well as through his errors. At times it can be a painful encounter also for the therapist, who may feel guilty about his own sometimes negative responses. Working through such feelings of guilt is part of the encounter.

The therapist's willingness to share with the patient that he has had experience with similar conflicts will often encourage a patient to cope with his pride or self-condemnation.

The mutually developing openness and the sharing of the patient's and therapist's humanness is the core of the healing process: Healing occurs because two people share in openness of their living and of their "being" with each other. In the process they both share judging each other, yet they share also the effort to understand each other. They share the struggle that goes with changing and with acceptance of the humanness that both will experience in each other. In this process the concept of an ideal world—the ideal self, ideal other people, ideal life in general—will become dissolved. The realistic experience of acceptance and tolerance and forgiving towards a nonperfect partner, leads ultimately towards the acceptance of the limitations of all life. This process must necessarily involve a resignation from the childhood dreams of perfection and omnipotence. Only this heals him from the hostility which grows out of disappointment. It moves him away from the idealizations of the past. He accepts the present reality as worthwhile, which protects him against frustrating disappointments. He will learn to accept himself and his partner, imperfect as they may be.

Healing communion will grow between patient and therapist when both have been able to communicate about their positive and negative feelings and have been able with each other mutually to accept their humanness and to accept each other. The self-inflicted isolation of the patient will cease; he will be able to be part of the human community. The therapist will also have gained in this relationship and doors will have opened up for him too. Each successful "encounter" will make the therapist a wiser therapist and person. Only then, when the patient as well as the therapist are on realistic grounds, when both can accept the inner polarity of love and hate in human hearts, can they (patient as well as the therapist) move towards their own lives, ready for new encounters and new unions—able to cope with temporary estrangement—ready to transcend this estrangement in never-ending struggle for communion.

When this stage is reached fully, therapy has reached its end and in some cases an enduring friendship will be born of a depth that is rare in our culture.

Here I should remind the reader that I have attempted to describe the "ideal type" of therapy, which is approximated in some cases, but, I fear, not in the average of the cases of an existential or any other therapist. With many patients the therapist will not reach the full depth of the encounter. Sometimes he will not be able to develop the degree of genuine affection which is needed for real closeness. In other cases the patient will be unable to overcome his fear of developing too deep a relationship. Often the therapist can help the patient beyond this anxiety, which is so common to man in our culture. At times some anxiety will remain and the relationship may come to an end with a sense of loss on both sides. In such cases some degree of success can still be achieved. The patient may be able to function somewhat better as a member of his family or in his work; some of his symptoms may disappear. Existential psychotherapy is no cure-all. It is not a "method" that can be learned by every therapist nor can it be successful with every patient. It is an approach which I believe gives a chance of success in many cases in which therapist and patient can find a common wavelength for communication.

Part II

In this part I will report a few episodes from my therapeutic practice which are selected to illustrate the various points made in the first part. I will describe a few examples in more detail hoping to give the reader a feeling of what goes on in a therapeutic hour.

1. *Initially the therapist struggles to find a common wavelength between himself and the patient, particularly if the therapist's first reaction is a negative one.*

Mrs.________ is a 59-year-old woman who came to me referred by a skin specialist. Diagnosis: lupus and arthritic-like side effects of the Cortisone drug—the Cortisone itself necessary to curb the lupus and at the same time to alleviate the arthritic pain. Both expected effects did not occur. This seemed unusual to her doctor. He sent her to me for investigating a possible emotional side to the unchanged severity of her situation.

Her anger seemed outrageous. She talked in an extremely low voice, enunciating each word slowly and beating her cane with each word on the couch which was next to her chair.

My reaction? I was appalled at the hard, controlled, and yet furious anger. I felt repulsed. The thought came that it would be more bearable if there was something more spontaneous in her fury—outbursts, tears, ups and downs in her voice. No, it was unpenetrable, stone.

At this point I wondered—could I bear to work with her? Was there any chance of ever penetrating the stoniness of her anger? Should I try to work with her? No. She would merely come to vent the anger; yet the massiveness of it would stay behind the stone wall of–defense? Yes, defense, I thought. But there was something else in her talking that began to touch me. I listened more closely with a grain more of willingness to feel with her: "She *causes* repulsion, and unconsciously needs to do so," I thought in the next hour. Both the drive to express her anger and to cause repulsion are balancing each other–she does not want to provoke sympathy–I felt. She provokes condemnation. Most people initially come for sympathy, pity, for being judged as "right." Not she.

She began at one of the hours, where I was already deeply involved in reading off my own reaction as to what possibly provoked her into the nearly frightening and powerful yet repulsive way of talking, when she with each cane-stroke on the couch summarized her inner situation as she saw it. I-am-full-of-the-most-vicious-hate-at-my-mother (who died so early)-at-my-sister,-who-took-care-of-me-and how!-at-my-father-who-was-looked-at-as-God-as-the-minister-of the-village-and-was-he-the-tyrant-of-the-house!-at-my-husband-who-is-a-spoiled-son-of-a-Yiddish-mama-and-wants-me-still to-serve-him,-me-in-this-condition,-stiff-all-swollen-all-raw,-at-the-doctor,-who-blows-me-up-with-Cortisone-and-it-does-not-help,-at-life,-which-gave-me-from-the-beginning-a-raw-deal,-and-at-God!!-?-who-treated-me-like-dirt.-All-these-sermons-about-grace-and-love,-God's love,-and-my love-? *I hate*.-?

She stopped. She had looked at me questioningly at intervals, producing repulsion, shock, yet also some sympathy, and looking, at the points most shocking to her, at me, how it would strike me. I could say at this point: "I admire your courage to face yourself. I admire that you can call hate hate, and don't want to pretend that you love, where no human being can possibly love."

I could respond with compassion that was reasoned out, but genuine. I had seen her profound despair, her honesty, and the abysmal condemnation of her hate. "That you dared to face your hate, even towards God, who did let this all happen to you–shows me the depth of your despair and of your lostness. But if you bring the picture of God into your anger, God is close. Maybe we have to work on a different concept about God and Life from that which your father had."

She then told me more about herself and her life. Her father had seemed like God at times, stern, severe, judging, demanding, and forgiving only if one repented. He looked like God to her and to other people too, and *they* admired him as they were moved to repentence by his powerful fundamentalist thunder of threats about hell. Not she, she hated God, who took her mother away when she was five, and hated her father, who demanded that she should take care of four younger siblings while an older but just as helpless and bossy sister had the supervision over her doings. She hated her sister who could handle the situation only by bossiness and tattling and cruelty and hate. It was too much for all. And their father demanded love or else hell. If one got sick, and only very sick, one got some care and warmth.

She raised the question all by herself, whether the untreatable sickness could be an outcome of her-54 years-of-accu-mu-la-ted hate and anger. "Do you think I got sick to get out of the rut of serving and serving spoiled Jack (her husband) and getting a little for myself? Yet I-did-not-get-anything-from-him.-I-hate-Jack-only-more." A self-punishment for all these years. The hate still going into her life now with Jack. And I added: "And a desperate cry for love and compassion in spite of your own hellish self-condemnation to eternal wrath." Her voice loosened up, she talked less deliberately, she fought with tears and then broke into tears.

I felt relief that suddenly there was a place where I could add a word that would touch and might begin to change her view of herself in this, her cruel world. I did not have to go into some sort of interpretation or explanation which would have meant to her merely preaching which she would not have believed and which she would have resented.

In many further hours I did feel growing compassion. I could help her accept her reaction of hate and despair with less terror and self-condemnation and accept life's limitations, that everybody had to come to terms with somehow. In the course of this work I could find in her quite tender places for other people's similar predicaments. Her own very barren childhood and the emptiness of life with Jack had made her go into painting—something for once for her. Selfish? "No! Just making something creative out of the barren and empty Cinderella feeling," I said. And she had given painting instruction to underprivileged children. I could again admire this spirit to transcend utter misery into some creativeness and creativeness for others.

And finally—hesitatingly—she confided in me her overpowering "need" for belonging to a church, her feeling that she did not deserve this belonging. She had insulted and thrown out her father's God. And I could say: "But your father's God is not necessarily the actual God, the ground of your—our being."

I changed over to my concept of God and she noticed it and was touched. It had a different sound from her father's God, who was so closely connected with hell. It made her question God from a new angle.

There was a very definite change in her physical reactions and the Cortisone began to have effect on the lupus and on the arthritis. She began to leave her cane in the waiting room—pretty soon at home.

She is not yet one with herself and does not yet accept fully the hateful side of herself. When her doctor, puzzled by the new physical reactions, suggested a checkup at one of the large hospitals in town, she again became very anxious and the new reactions disappeared. She was scared of all the tests which made her furious, and she was scared of possibly having to talk with someone again who might not be sympathetic to her hate.

The description of the beginning of my work with this woman shows clearly the process on my side—a slow progress from the disgust and even fear that I found in myself to more and more recognition of what else was touched off in me. I experienced a gradual change towards understanding and finally found a place where I could make her feel the condition which caused her fierce condemnation. This, I believe, resulted from the fact that I could genuinely admire the integrity of her not pretending love, and of her not conforming with the most essential demand of the father's wrathful threats of hell, to love where she could not.

2. *In my second example, early in treatment a situation arises which is puzzling, both to the patient and me. Such an occurrence could endanger the development of a relationship, or, if clarified, could become an important event in the development of true "encounter." It may help in the clarification of the relationshp if both patient and therapist express what they associate with the "event." By searching for the validity of the association, the event may be further clarified and a positive encounter may be engendered.*

An episode with Martin illustrates a case of sharing genuine reactions on both sides.

Martin is a young man who grew up as a twin to a sister who was obviously preferred, and as all women in his family were, was regarded as "stronger and better" than the men. He had been in analysis before in New York and, in the beginning, he wanted only to sketch his family relations. He would fill in missing parts later. It was striking that he completely avoided talking about his twin sister—a very important part of his life. When I felt I needed to know at least something about the relationship that existed between Lois and him, there was silence for a whole hour. Next time he brought an album of photographs along. This hour also passed in silence. I was puzzled, felt increasingly uncomfortable. When I expressed that I felt in some ways pushed away he objected. "My feeling is rather the opposite," he said. "Puzzling way of expressing the opposite (of pushing me away)," I responded. He could not understand my feeling and insisted on his disagreement. My mind went to the Japanese custom of long silence when one visits one of the Zen masters. This always had felt to me like time granted to slowly abandoning the things of the past that occupy one's mind and a slow turning to the present experience, to an opening up and meeting of *this* person. Thinking of this and mentioning it, I tried to turn more to *him* and I glanced through the album. The silence ceased to be uncomfortable for me and what I saw now in some of the family pictures was indeed an important message: an overwhelming show of togetherness, sameness in dress and toys, as well as a show of the overwhelming work which these two babies must have caused. The album began to carry its message to my mind. After a while I verbalized my impression of the pictures, but there was still no response to it from my patient—rather a more stony silence. I dropped further questions about the album. I observed at this time the double circle he endlessly drew with a finger of his right hand ○○. I saw his strong piano hand (he had studied the piano and had won, as the first prize, a scholarship; his sister had won the second prize in the same contest; and because of this he was not permitted to accept the scholarship. His parents could not allow either of the twins to be ahead of the other). I observed an urge in me to touch the hand of him, who seemed to slide more and more away from me and from reality. (Countertransference: His hand reminded me of the hand of the brother of my first childhood boyfriend, with whom I had played four-hand pieces on the piano while my boyfriend was, for health reasons, away in a boarding school.) I *did*, shortly, touch his hand in an attempt to reach him, the way a child therapist does with a withdrawing child. I found the utterly soft hand of an infant and I understood intuitively: He was caught in the conflict of wanting to be like an infant to me and wanting me alone to himself without his sister Lois and without talk about her. This was a paralyzing conflict—she felt like a part of him. There was his conflict: I should not have any knowledge of Lois and still he was so close to Lois: ○○. On the pre-verbal level he was silent when I asked him about Lois *and* his finger drew the symbol for the closeness incessantly: His associations to ○○ were the rubbing of twins in the womb.

In working on this experience between us, he expressed that he felt that my touching his hand had given me a shock and some disappointment. I said: "Yes, I feel you are right, it was a surprise not to find the strong piano hand I saw and expected. Instead of the hand similar to that of a childhood friend, I felt the hand of a little helpless infant who wants and needs a mother all alone, to himself. I was rather glad to have found the explanation for your puzzling statement: 'It's rather the opposite to pushing you away.' "

Another episode from my work with Martin relates to a visit with his parents over a weekend. He was full of disgust about his father's routine before dinner, moaning and groaning about his duty to serve.

He did this especially when guests were invited and his mother had put a great deal of effort into the preparation of dinner. Martin's sister objected openly to this rather offensive moaning while Martin frantically tried to divert from it by making friendly conversation with the guests. He was seething inside with hate but covered up the rudeness of his father. I reacted quite spontaneously to his covering up efforts, saying, "You know, I hate that kind of pussy-footing, covering up of an angry situtation. I think Lois was quite courageous in saying something in the open." He repeated my word, "hate–hate: You hate me."

I began to become defensive, "It was just a way of saying that I would rather have feelings outspoken than covered up. I did not mean that I hate *you*." "No," he said, "these are excuses, you hate 'this' and 'this' means me." I responded, "I know, you mean I behave like the nursery school teacher who says: 'I hate what you are doing, but not you, of course.' " "Yes," he said, "that's exactly it. You hate me." He described more of his sinking feeling. He did not want to accept any of my explanations of the expression "I hate it." I felt pinned down, cornered. I did not hate him. I felt I had carelessly used this word, yet he sank and sank. I became depressed. After all, the regular, traditional analytic method would have been less destructive. I should have sized up the situation as more vulnerable than I apparently had spontaneously thought of it.

I finally said, "I don't think we can clarify anything at this point. Let's start anew next time and stop now, as painful as the present situation is for both of us."

He left. I myself had a sunken feeling. The incident went with me for the next two days and I still felt that the "hate" I had expressed was so temporary, so light, that it actually could barely be called hate. In these two days I began to feel what he actually must have experienced at home. It dawned on me that there must have been a hate of his very existence of a dimension that was practically unknown to me so far.

When I had corrected the word hate that evening to "irritation" he only got into more despair. This was what his mother and also his father had done. They let him feel utterly exasperated by hate and then became guilty and changed the word into something less guilty. Still, he felt the first word "hate" was what his parents actually had felt. That was why he could not accept any of my efforts to correct the word "hate."

The mother–immature herself–suddenly had two babies. When they expected the afterbirth to come, it was instead, Martin. His father left his mother alone for four months after the twins were born–there was litte attention for Martin in the home. The mother stayed with the father's family, unwanted amidst a large family of aunts and the grandmother, nobody helping her but indicating how much of a nuisance the continually crying infants were to the family. Hate around, abysmally deep, coming out of despair at not being able to cope with the "too much" of the situation which nobody had wanted or planned. Hate for the babies, especially for the second one, the surprise, the "afterbirth." The photo album came into my mind—every picture stressing the "too much," yet at the same time making it look like joy, phony joy. The hate of it had to be turned into love but Martin was familiar from his very early months with the unexpressed hate underneath. His mother could, at times, talk in the past tense of the hate; his father talked in not misunderstandable terms of how awful it all had always been.

When at the next hour I suggested that I wondered whether it was this old hate that had been touched in the last hour, a hate I had not ever experienced, Martin said: "This I can accept. This must be true. I believe you, that your 'I hate it' was not the hate I know."

He now began to say that he had on his side, for two days, a time of rage against me, continuing rage, rage, hate, fury, rage. He had hoped to express it to me, he had planned to express it to me, but when he saw me now he had known immediately that it did not really belong to me.

There had been a strange ending of his rage the night before he came to me again. He had worried whether I would become more cautious and controlled after the last hour. Now he was relieved that I did not seem to be inhibited. He felt puzzled that he had not ever been able to say my name in any form whatsoever. He had tried to understand it. But he still could not accept the interpretation I had given that I was not yet a real person but a "therapist" for him. Rather the opposite he felt was true: I was the only person at this point who felt real and spontaneous to him. And now after this "encounter" at the end of his rage, he could rather tenderly say, "Good night, Hanna Colm, good night." For the first time that night he had mentioned my name, even though only to himself.

He searched the next morning, where the melody, the rhythm of "Good night, Hanna Colm, good night" belonged, and with the help of a colleague, he had found that it was of the theme song in The Music Man—rather on the romantic side.

He was puzzled. I, not as much when he told me the next day. The hate was expressed and out of his system for the time being; now there was place for tenderness he also felt towards me. It was an experience he never had had before—that hate and love can be going on in a person at the same time and also that hate can be temporary—not final—as love can be fluctuating in all human beings. He was afraid of this "flicker of a flame of tenderness"–"it had also a killing potential," he ventured. He could not say as yet whether this touched off the love with which his mother had always had to cover up her "hate of it." He rather felt that he was deadly scared of tender feelings–disappointment?–too overwhelming in his need for tenderness.

He brought the words of the theme song of The Music Man, which touched something in me, dreams of "someone" going to "someone." It was interesting, this namelessness in the song–"Good night, my someone, Good night:" The whole song provoked in me old memories of my early teens, longing for someone, sweet, romantic, far off, really unreal, yet the first sweet inkling of "someone" who would respond and to whom one would respond.

When he, an hour later, also brought the record with a picture of a young boy floating through the air with a young girl, it became clear to me, that I should not take this "Good night, Hanna Colm, good night" as demonstrating real tenderness and affection. It was, as the memories which the song stirred up, a very young teenager's longings for love and being loved. But there was not yet really experienced affection in this song. Yet the longing was already a first step into affection.

I told him how the words of the song and the record had impressed me, what they had touched off in me first and that they finally made clear to me that they had too much unrealistic idealism in the mood of the words, that he and I should be aware of it; maybe that what really went on between us with all its fluctuations from real hate to tenderness, from disagreement to real union of thought and feeling was actually already more tenderness or affection than this song protrayed.

He was grateful that I had made this point, especially as he felt that his mother rather had this super-idealistic view about "love," which seemed to him actually to be utterly unrealistic and the cause of endless disappointment.

Another episode with Martin: Martin had recently gotten again into a period of silence. Here it was again, this time in horror of what a scene in the bathroom had done to him as a child. An hour before he had told me how his twin sister and he used to sit in the bathtub, watching his mother at the sink, one leg in it, shaving her hair off ("hair was disgusting to her"), often bleeding also. He did not know why, but he saw it with horror. "People are different. She seemed to have disgust of hair. I, for instance, like hair," I said.

He could not talk after this story, the next time. I wondered what would shut him off, and ventured with my own associations about this scene: I saw something positive about hair. "Hair was disgusting to her, she feels different about hair than I feel. How do *you* feel about the hair on your hands, arms, chest?" His response: "Yes, indeed, I never knew hair *was* disgusting to her—my God—that's why so often I feel the urge to shave all hair off before I stage the fights." Martin had to stage fights in fantasy and with furniture when he was depressed or disgusted with himself.

A memory came up in Martin—long forgotten—that indeed the first physical fights happened in the bathroom with Lois on top of him. He always had to let her be first, to win (we had talked about this before). Silence—more silence. I had my own associations, with a damp hot bathroom I told him about this. Then he said: "I *feel* it again—I *feel* it; the dampness, the hotness. That's why I imagine any love being sweaty, damp, wet in my fighting, a thing which I loathe in real life." And from here his associations did begin to flow easily and did bring up a great number of pushed-out-of-sight feelings, what these fighting scenes meant to him.

At times the patient might reject completely the therapist's associations which are suggested to him. Then the therapist must be willing to admit that her own associations may not be applicable to the patient. This easy admission can be of importance to the patient, seeing that the therapist does not need always to be right and does not want to be taken merely as an authority. When a rejection is given *too* violently, I might say, "let's give it a chance and sleep over it for a night or two. Your intensity suggests a bit that my association must have touched off something in you." Often the patient comes back with it later in a slightly different form. When none of the therapist's suggestions are accepted by the patient, this might have to be studied. Martin for hours denied whatever I ventured for a further understanding of his imagined fights. I felt utterly useless—nearly impotent, and the association of Martin's father's threat to castrate him, to cut his sister's breasts off, came to my mind. I told him this association. I reminded him that he himself felt that great envy was involved in his father's threats. I wondered now whether there was possibly envy involved towards me, envy which would signify then a meaningless competition between us and the need to negate whatever I would say. I wondered whether envy was involved in his relation to all women, and this in conflict with his *need* for them (closeness to Lois *and* envy: she did not have disgusting hair, and so on). This clicked. Envy that always has to destroy or render omnipotent the envied one. This hit home. Our work came to life again.

3. *The therapist expresses his negative feelings about a patient:*

description of the therapist's struggle with negative feelings when there is a basically positively experienced relationship. Several examples may illustrate this situation.

A patient who was working on her need to placate with "goody-goody" performances had great difficulty to look at herself and what was behind her goodness and her conforming. She began after a while to condemn her placating and I felt this was not really working seriously on her problem. One day I simply said: "You *bore* me with both the self-citation of your goodness and your utter self-condemnation." Only with this expression of strong feelings did she turn to the "why" of her goodness and her self-condemnation at the same time. I could say this "You bore me" only after I also did feel quite strongly with her and about her.

Another example is a young minister, very unsure of himself, who also played the "goody-goody" all his life. I felt so relieved when he dared to question his goodness and even suspect his homosexuality as his very private attempt to be bad once in a while. I ventured, "Thank God, you did dare at least secretly to be bad and experiment with life beyond merely conforming with your mother's standards. But you couldn't quite get through with it and ended up again with the pursuit of the ideal of yourself in your homosexual fantasies also. That is too bad!"

Another person compared himself endlessly with his stepfather, his brother, and uncle–practically with every man and never could find anybody who was not by far superior to him. He ought to have been this way or that, but he was not. I finally responded quite impatiently with "Who do you think you really are? This constant comparing with others and running yourself down. It slowly but surely gets me, what is it all about?" We found, only now after my expression of impatience, that after he lost his father at three, this father became more and more an ideal to him, as did a sister who died later. He desperately competed for his mother with his stepfather and uncle, who on their side also competed then for his dependent forlorn mother, yet he of course could never make it. He was handicapped by the tabu of competing for a mother, so the comparison turned out to be an endless running himself down.

4. *The patient who attacks a countertransference in the therapist and the therapist accepts his help: cooperative search about both partners' feelings.*

Paul, a young minister who was a year out of his job, because of stagefright, was installed again as a minister in one of the rather big churches. The celebration to which he invited me was quite ceremonial and impressive. An old teacher of his, to whom he felt he owed a great deal had agreed to give the sermon for his installation. The sermon was given in such exaggerated mannerism, nearly theatrical in gesture and speech, that I had trouble to listen. I read the sermon later—it was an extraordinarily good one, yet the manner of presentation repulsed me, it evoked my own problem of hating phony performances—my own father had been a minister and was so often phony, though in rather a different way, that I invariably not only rejected phoniness violently but also invariably responded to it with a rather blunt frankness about it.

When we went in line to congratulate this young minister, my husband, who was also invited for the occasion, knowing me, suggested: "Say something nice, it's a very important day for him and he is very devoted to his teacher." Yet, I could not. I shook hands, congratulated him and said nothing about the sermon.

My patient, then on the way not to be my patient much longer, came to his next hour asking, "You did not say anything about my teacher's simply great sermon?" I told him that I had not been able to listen too much. "His manner of making a great show of gestures had distracted me. Gerhard, though, had been able to listen in spite of it, and found it indeed great in content. I know I have a problem about phoniness not yet worked out. I still seem to want nothing of a presentation if the person indulges in his oratory as much as your teacher did." Whereupon Paul, somewhat disappointed, very modestly, but rather tolerantly said: "Do you always know when *you* are phony? I think, nobody really can know but God. Your reaction to it seems rather righteous and without love, and *that* is the ultimate value." He was right.

Paul's quiet reproach hit home and ever since has liberated me from the feeling—"only not be phony." Both my husband's and his words said unspokenly—there is a higher value than not ever being phony—understanding, tolerance, and in this particular situation, the affection for Paul, which I did deeply have, but which was pushed out of sight by my own problem about phoniness.

5. *Not only the patient but also the therapist may express tender feelings, but tender feelings might touch off struggle and anxiety in the patient.*

Gladys will have to leave in a few weeks on Peace Corps work in the Near East. She has talked over with me that she will have to take indoctrination classes besides packing up the household here and will have to stop therapy four to five weeks earlier than she would otherwise need. I had the feeling that we still had ten days or two weeks left when she worked on the feeling that ending earlier than absolutely necessary did feel harder and nearly unbearable. She felt like crying—and felt suddenly "silly" to have planned the early ending even though it was sensible. At the end of the hour she got up with the conclusion to go through with the early ending in order not to get into her old problem of taking on too much and resenting it then in a sort of martyr attitude. She suddenly hugged me in tears and kissed me. I responded, also touched to tears: "How nice to show me your affection now when it welled up in you and not only in a few weeks when you leave." Whereupon she said "This is the last hour. Did you forget?" "Yes, I did push it out of sight, Gladys–too painful"–and I took her back again for another good-by hug. She left–"I am overjoyed that it is you who forgot it, Hanna!"

A very human defense experienced in the "therapist" which added to the depth of the expression of feeling between both of us. She had ceased to be a patient.

A young woman had to deny affection and dependency–her father had died suddenly in a plane crash, her mother had committed suicide, but she acted out dependency and helplessness. She had to be indecisive in every little or big situation which called for a decision. This served also as an unconscious means to annoy the people around her–to keep them off. She would not ever be involved with anybody again, she would rather play with suicide herself if her self-defeating loneliness became too desperate.

She had felt unloved all her life–her defense, "I don't want ever to care again," had only developed to a climax when she lost her parents in short succession. The reaction to the sudden death of both parents was in a way a rationalization and confirmation of her life-long defense: "I don't care whether I am loved, I rather annoy everybody, I don't want ever to feel too much. I don't even assume somebody ever could love me. I annoy everybody and make sure nobody really wants me."

I had a dream about Bertha, born out of frustration. I dreamed that she was talking to another woman who sat on the edge of the couch on which she was lying. And I clearly heard Bertha say to her "She loves me, I know it, Hanna really loves me." I was touched to tears in the dream and relieved of the deep frustration into which she had led me with her–"I don't ever really care, nobody loves me, I don't ever believe it, I don't ever want any love. But I do have the power to upset everybody instead."

According to recent literature on countertransference[1] a dream of an analyst about his patient indicates an emotional involvement within himself. The analyst should become aware of it and should try to overcome it.

I knew also from my own inner feeling, that this dream was a very human and positive and real reaction to Bertha's defensive "I don't

1. Mabel Cohen, *Psychiatry*, "Counter-Transference and Anxiety," Vol. 15, pp. 231-243 (1952).

care." It demonstrated that I had felt hurt as had other people around her who had compassion and affection for her and were so thoroughly frustrated, rejected, and defeated by her. My own reaction in the dream—"My God, she cares!" made me aware *how* much I felt frustrated and how much I cared in compassion and affection for her "in spite."

I decided to share with her this dream and to work out with her all the potential reactions which this sharing would indicate in her and in me.

Bertha listened and did not say the expected "Oh, I don't really want to hear this, I don't really care." She said, instead, in tears, "How sweet of you, how incredible that you could tell me of such intimate and tender feelings, with the chance that I would just reject you again." And this little event started off quite a long time of working on some, up to now, undiscovered factors of Bertha's "I don't care." She could look at her continued envy of a younger brother, who was preferred to her, the envy which made her feel she had not gotten much, which made her resent what others had, and which made her first defeat them and then punish herself with feelings of worthlessness, guilt, and loneliness.

My unconscious declaration of my need for reassurance and my caring was convincing to her, while a verbal declaration of my affection, I am sure, would not have convinced her; she would not have believed it.

I asked myself whether I would have shared a negative dream with a patient. It is hard to answer this in the abstract. But I know it would depend on the special time of the therapeutic process at which it would occur and on the depth of positive relationship that had already developed. In the very beginning of the developing relationship, I would not share a negative, maybe also not a positive dream; it would depend on the situation. Patients are at the beginning often too scared of negative as well as positive feelings. If a relationship of some depth had developed and a negative dream would show a feeling that naturally, at times, comes up in the very complex process of "encounter," I would dare to share it and work towards a mutual acceptance of the possibility of the nonexclusive presence of positive *and* negative feelings.

6. *The therapist may at times share his own past and present struggle with the conflict with which the patient struggles.*

I had Harry, 8, with me, whose envy of his sister, of girls, was obvious and unacceptable to him, partially because it is scary for a boy to really want to be a girl and in the process have to get rid of "something" which really is part of him and which he does not really want to part with.

He drew a number of "important men"—he also envied the importance of his father "who even talked at times to the President," but it was obvious that all these important men whom he drew had hair-dos like girls. He could smile a little sheepishly when I made a remark about his important father, but as he kept drawing these particular men with girl's hair-dos—George Washington, Thomas Jefferson—I once carefully asked him whether he did not feel at times a bit angry that he could not be, as yet, as important as Dad was and could not even have all the fancy hair-dos and everything else that his sister had in addition to what he had: Did he want to be a man with a sort of girl's hair-do? He denied it flatly—no smile—oh, no, he never would. Only when I told him about myself as a kid of his age and how envious I was of my little brother, did he smile and ask me: "What did you do then?" "Oh," I said, "I first just was very envious here and there, but then I thought when he did not do well in school, I could out-do him! I really could and then when I was all grown up and came to this country and all the women wore slacks I thought "Now I can be a woman and wear slacks—ha!" He had a big smile now and said: "That's why I like to draw these men with the hair-dos." I said, I know—I knew also he had a harder trouble than I had—to be a bit envious of little sisters must feel sissyish or babyish, with all his baby sisters. *I* as a kid could simply be a bit of a tomboy and everybody thought only that that was sort of cute.

Harry had also deep conflicts about growing up, wanting both to stay dependent and to be important and big. When he had his last hour, because his parents planned to leave the country for a job in Africa, he drew first a lion, an angry and dangerous-looking one, and wanted to take that picture home for himself. He drew bars in front of the lion and then, for me also drew a baby deer eating from a green bush, "See, it's a baby deer?" "Yes," I said, "a dear baby!" He smiled at me and said "You really love me." "Yes," I replied, "I do, just the way you are—there is in you a big lion, the King of the animals, but behind bars and not dangerous any more, and there is in you a baby deer also." And he replied: "I love you, too." "I feel it," I replied, "even though you know about me and my brother."

He cried bitterly all the way home from the last hour—he could let himself feel the grief of separation and could show it also to his mother, who drove him. He was sure and could trust at this moment that two people could love him and not laugh at his tears, and he could love two people, without the haunting doubts of envy. He was sure that neither I nor his mother nor he himself would feel he was simply sissyish or whiny. No, he also accepted the baby-deer side of himself. He summarized, when he arrived home, in the midst of tears: "And I am still looking forward to going to Africa." What an acceptance of conflicting feelings!—expressed in the space of one hour. Even though he has finished treatment prematurely, because of his father's new job, there will remain in Harry many more two-way feelings, but I am sure, he will make it all right.

Of course, one has to size up the importance to the patient of personal reactions, sharing associations, and the answers of the therapist, but also in which phase of the treatment the patient is—can he keep an intimate answer for himself, or will he use it in a hostile way. This will depend widely on two factors: First, *when* questions like this are asked, *how much* hostility is already worked out and *how much* is he already struggling to feel like a real partner to the therapist; and second, how self-acceptant the therapist himself is and how dependent still on an ideal concept about himself. He might then frankly say, "I am still touchy in this area and cannot really answer your question comfortably." Or, "This question actually is so complicated to answer that I cannot comfortably answer it in a short yes or no way, it would distract us from our work too long." Still, both answers suggest that the therapist has struggled also in this area and does not try to create an ideal image about himself. And not only this fact is important in his answer, but also that he has a right to his privacy and to a denial, not to distract the work on the problems of this patient for too long, when a short answer would distort his communication.

In the process of the therapeutic encounter between the patient and the therapist, both try to liberate the patient from his "conforming rebellion;" both try to find the point in the patient's symptoms in which his rebellion conveys a basic integrity, yet where he did not really become alive to the present and free himself from a past authority.

The therapist participating in the patient's "conforming rebellion" can help him experience where his rebellion and where his secret conforming do not allow him to be one with himself, where the unresolved past secretly still interferes with the fully *present* living of the patient, and where old defenses prevent him from taking the risks of a genuine relationship, and thus can help him actually to be himself.

In the open communion of the therapeutic encounter the therapist is alerted to the patient's attempts at integrity and to his failures to achieve it by clinging to the past and by defenses that once were necessary but may not be needed any more. The life of the patient is reevaluated in terms of genuineness as to its presentness and lack of no longer necessary defenses. And as the relationship grows the patient becomes just as alerted to the therapist's integrity in spite of left-over human clinging to the safety of the past and to its defenses. Now both help each other in growing towards genuine living.

It is essential that the patient can share the therapist's own feelings, his associations evoked by a patient's problem, his dreams at times, or his countertransferences. Then he will, in the framework of therapy as encounter, experience how seriously the therapist takes his partnership and the feelings and reactions he brings into the partnership. Encounter reveals itself as a slowly developing process on both sides, which centers around the patient's needs especially in the beginning, but then slowly develops into a genuine relationship, with growth on both sides.

This slowly growing relationship starts out on both sides with caution: Cautious carefulness on the side of the therapist and caution and even suspicion on the side of the patient. This caution develops into greater trust and potentially greater and greater sharing of both participants' humanness and willingness to work conflicts through towards ever-renewed genuine interaction.

The therapist's expression of his reactions and even of his irrational countertransference makes for far shorter periods of regression in the patient. Regression does appear, yet is worked through faster. It makes the therapeutic experience less frustrated by loneliness; it helps to overcome withdrawal and to accept a realistic polaric positive-negative relationship; it makes possible a no longer so frightening experience in closeness, which then in turn soon becomes the focus of the clarifying encounter.

Growth towards reality is achieved faster through the experience of genuineness than through an experience of prescribed frustration which the Freudian unresponsive and unqualified acceptance may actually create.

This process is often a painful one, because it involves throwing away past securities, past and present defenses, and idealized concepts of oneself and one's partner, and acceptance of oneself and of one's partner in mutual humanness—"in spite" of and with the human predicaments with which both struggle.

The closeness, which will remain between patient and therapist, will eventually be that of two friends, who now do not any longer need to see each other at regular intervals. They see each other when both feel like it and when conditions permit it.

Sometimes the ways of patient and therapist do not cross again any longer for various reasons, but sometimes they can meet occasionally and then it feels like a gift of grace if the center-contact has stayed alive and can be immediately re-established without one-sided dependency but in a dependency on each other and in mutual openness towards each other, which leaves the friend, whom one helped to grow and through whom one grew oneself, free in communion and trust.[2]

2. To show how a patient experienced the Therapeutic Encounter I quote from a letter received after the author's death: "Riding up on the plane to Washington, I kept remembering . . . her willingness to sacrifice psychoanalytic orthodoxy in order to share with me, her patient, her own fears and deep concerns, for she believed that only by a sharing in self-giving, only by love, could any true healing take place–her passionate concern to find what she called the 'wholesome' or what I would call 'religious truth' . . . the candle expressed her life–it exhausted itself in giving out warmth and light." [Ed.]

18

EDITH WEIGERT

The Importance of Flexibility in Psychoanalytic Technique

Psychoanalytic science has grown out of an art, Freud's art of investigating and treating psychoneurotic patients. The scientific discoveries of the dynamic unconscious, of the steps of human libido development, of repression, regression, transference, repetition compulsion, etc., have in turn influenced the art of psychoanalytic practice. Psychoanalytic practitioners, the artists in this profession, remain the pioneering vanguard of psychoanalytic science. The scientists follow them, consolidating their intuitive discoveries and conquests. Such a vanguard has to be flexible and mobile, not to get frozen in what Freud called "the pseudo exactness of modern psychiatry."

The technique of psychoanalytic art is built on a set of rules or suggestions for practical procedures which cannot in the least cover the almost infinite variety of therapeutic situations arising in analysis, which Freud compared with the complex constellations of a chess game. Freud, in his papers on technique, as well as Ella Sharpe, Fenichel, Glover, Strachey and other early authors who wrote on technique have stressed the need for flexibility for various reasons:

(1) Freud emphasized that his technical suggestions were suited to his individuality and that another personality might be led to a different attitude toward the patient and the therapeutic task. This remark shows Freud's respect for differences in technical style. The unconscious of the analyst is a receiving organ. His countertransference, lifted into consciousness, becomes an important source of

Reprinted with permission of the pbulisher from the *Journal of the American Psychoanalytic Association*, 1954, Vol. 2, 702-710 information in the analytic process. Any rigidity, any automatization of attitude or procedure can become a defense against intuitive insight and block the passage from the unconscious to the conscious processes of the analyst. It is therefore important that the spontaneity of the psychoanalyst not be muffled by the rigidity of his technique.

(2) In 1918 Freud said: "Different forms of illness which we treat cannot be handled with the same form of technique." The treatment of hysteria differs from that of a phobia or that of an obsessional neurosis. Since that time analytic treatment has spread out beyond the field of the typical neuroses. Nowadays it is even sometimes difficult to pick typical psychoneuroses for teaching and training purposes since there are more atypical character neuroses seeking treatment. Psychoanalytic treatment has come to encompass children, adolescents, persons in the advanced age group, character neuroses with difficulties of adjustment in marriage, family or work relations, psychosomatic diseases, psychopathic conditions and borderline cases. The functional psychoses or narcissistic neuroses have been tackled, proving Freud's original thesis that loss of reality and corresponding shrinkage of the ego are only quantitatively, not qualitatively different in psychoses and neuroses. A great differentiation of technique became necessary to do justice to the variations of therapeutic needs of all these patients newly admitted to psychoanalytic treatment.

(3) A third source of change in technique stems from the very development of psychoanalytic science during the lifetime of Freud and thereafter. For instance, the change in the concept of anxiety has provided us with a new searchlight not only into libidinal repressions, but also into inhibitions and distortions of aggression and their influence on the pregenital as well as oedipal stages of libido development. Our new insight into the structure of psychoses has enriched our knowledge about the early development in neuroses. The narcissistic withdrawal into fantastic grandiosity and magic manipulations which seemed originally inaccessible to transference interpretations has entered into the orbit of psychoanalytic treatment. A much more detailed knowledge of the ego and its defenses has intensified our resistance analysis and more and more prevented a premature, intellectualized communication of unconscious contents, before the resistances have been "melted in the fire of transference." In navigating between what Fenichel called the "Scylla and Charybdis of psychoanalytic technique"—the resistance of acting out and that of intellectualization—we find that the resistance of intellectualization has increased with the growing popularity of psychoanalysis. Sophisticated patients use technical terms without emotional partici-

pation. We have increasingly to insist that the patient express himself in plain English, which is closer to his emotions.

The rapid growth of psychoanalysis and its popularization contain other dangers. Freud has predicated that the spreading of psychoanalytic therapy would lead to the gold of analysis being alloyed with the copper of a psychotherapy working with suggestion and re-education. We find it difficult to draw the line between psychoanalysis and psychotherapy. For instance, the modification of the patient's superego, a precondition for further change, the mitigation of superego rigidity, is accomplished by the personal influence of the analyst as "auxiliary superego" in early stages of analysis. This is a form of re-education. The borderline between nondirective interpretation and directive re-education is fluid. We have become more aware of the elements of reality estrangement and ego shrinkage in character neuroses, and realize that these infantile elements need re-education as well as analysis, just as children need this combination, according to Anna Freud. In the infantile arrested ego there are gaps of alienation from reality loaded with anxiety.

The pillars in the edifice of psychoanalytic technique are the elucidation of resistance and transference. In recent papers by Gitelson, Whittacker, Paula Heiman, Annie Reich, Buxbaum, Mabel Cohen and others there is a growing emphasis on the importance of lifting countertransference into the consciousness of the analyst, not for communication to the patient, but in order to improve and refine the standards of the work. The most thorough analytic elucidation of resistance, transference and countertransference is the essential criterion of value in the psychoanalytic work. Granted, it is not easy to assess the management of resistance, transference, and countertransference in the intricacies of another analyst's therapeutic activities. If, instead of the study of microscopic findings in the analytic workshop, we use the microscopic criterion of adherence to certain rules, our judgment might easily be misled, since adherence to rules can be the expression of an unanalytic rigidity. I agree with what Fenichel said about technical rules:

> The observance of a prescribed ceremonial produces a magical impression and may be misinterpreted by the patient in this sense. We know . . . that we can and must be elastic in the application of all technical rules. Everything is permissible, if only one knows why. Not external measures, but the management of resistance and transference is the criterion whether a procedure is analysis or not.

Let us look more closely at some of the rules on which psychoanalytic technique is based. The fundamental rule of free associations represents an ideal of spontaneous freedom, conducive to the revelation of the unconscious. But this ideal is only approximated in advanced stages of successful analysis. The manifold individual deviations from the fundamental rule are grist to the analytic mill. Analysis lives on resistance. The ways in which each patient circumvents the basic rule, by halting, silence, rambling, obscurities, etc., deliver important information about individual resistances and instinct derivatives. The basic rule cannot be enforced. The rule about "no major decisions" also has to be handled with flexibility, otherwise patients who are inclined to act out would discontinue prematurely, or a patient who is well enough progressed to make such decision might hide his ability to take responsibilities behind the defense of literal obedience to the rule.

The rule about the reclining position has, according to Freud, historical reasons (development of analysis out of hypnosis). The position of the analyst out of sight of the analysand was a convenience personally agreeable to Freud. It has the disadvantage that the analyst cannot observe the facial expression of the analysand. If this rule is used with flexibility, the patient being permitted to change his position, he may reveal therewith defenses or impulsive derivatives. In any case, it is important to analyze the magic implications of this and other rules, which the patient accepts as conventionalities in submission or rebellion.

Since Alexander and his collaborators have introduced their well-known experiments in "psychoanalytic therapy," the rule about frequency of analytic interviews has particularly stirred up clouds of distrust and alienation among analysts—a reaction which seems to me contrary to the spirit of psychoanalysis and the intimacy of mutual understanding. Freud saw his patients six times weekly; lighter cases and more progressed patients were seen three times weekly. This arrangement was obviously adjusted to the Central European working week, which did not include the long week end of the Anglo-Saxon British and Americans. The "Monday crust" that Freud described in those patients whom he saw six times weekly is often a phenomenon of resistance, a reaction formation against frustrated dependency needs. Similar resistances cannot, and need not, be avoided. They may throw dependency, separation anxieties, reactions of grief or rage into relief which might go undiscovered or be delayed in their access to insight when an instituted frequency rule has become a habit on which the patient relies automatically. The spirit of the rule that analysis has to be carried out in abstinence, specifically in abstinence of infantile satisfactions, may be violated by a rigidly maintained frequency rule. A patient with a weak ego and rarefied reality relations may develop an addiction to analysis which can form a defensive armor, harder to pierce than the Monday crust of the typical psychoneurotic.

It is obvious that the development of transference needs a steadfast continuity in the relation between analyst and analysand. But the rhythm of this continutiy varies from patient to patient and in different phases of analysis. In severe panic states even daily interviews are not sufficient to maintain a continuity of relation. Hospitalization may become necessary and distribution of transference over a continuously available rotating hospital staff occurs. The degree of free-floating anxieties which are no longer or not yet crystallized in defenses is a means of determining the optimal frequency of psychoanalytic hours at a certain period of analysis. If anxieties and therewith libido cannot be sufficiently mobilized, the most religious maintenance of daily interviews does not break through the defensive armor and a classical form of analysis cannot yet be established. For instance, a very withdrawn, schizoid obsessional character felt so threatened by the closeness of daily interviews that he increased his defenses of indifference and boredom which made him more unreachable.

A certain differentiation in frequency often seems useful in a character neurosis with pregenital fixations. I think here of a type of schizoid patient who nowadays frequently seeks treatment, who does not so much suffer from acute symptoms due to actualized conflict but from emotional immaturity, partial withdrawal from reality and vague anxieties about a possible psychotic break. Such a patient has often a good intellectual grasp of his difficulties, describing them in analytical terms but without living through their emotional impact. When this patient talks rather glibly about his castration anxieties, his fears of incorporating or being swallowed up, this does not indicate an untamable id strength that floods the ego with unconscious material, but an estranged aloofness from inner as well as outer reality which splits the weak ego into a rather cynical observer and a more or less unstable actor. In the schizoid patient the observer keeps the upper hand. This split in the schizoid patient is very different from the therapeutic split in the acutely regressed neurotic patient described by Sterba which is most helpful when the patient had partially reached the genital level before. As long as the pregenital fixations prevail due to early arrest of libidinal development, the split remains untherapeutic, the power of integration is poor, the sublimations are unstable and the patient is inclined to fill his inner emptiness by making out of analysis a pseudo religion and to establish an addicted transference. The ambivalence of this transference is neutralized in dependency ingeniously disguised, since the schizoid patient is attracted to and deadly afraid of this dependency. Such a patient said to me after a long period of daily interviews: "I do not dare to work wholeheartedly outside of analysis, since I feel compelled to remain completely absorbed in analysis." In this case, in which I was consulted, a change from five to three weekly hours was suggested and the masochistic transference became accessible to analysis. The patient recognized that he had tried to achieve a magical cure by absorption in analysis. His work inhibition decreased while he dared more to experiment on the outside.

We have found it useful to spread the analysis of a schizoid patient out over a longer period of time in which the transference, and particularly the pregenital character of transference, remains exposed to analysis. The analyst is at the patient's disposal for intensified treatment whenever an emergency or unusual stress occurs. But the maturing process needs time and gradual increase of realistic experiences so that the patient can catch up with the gaps in his libidinal development. He needs to test out his gains from the protected analytic experience in his less protected extra-analytic relations. When the analyst succeeds in eliciting trust in the patient on the basis of an aim-inhibited libidinal attachment, the split in the schizoid patient becomes truly therapeutic, his integration becomes more stabilized, his sublimations spread out. The intuition and the tact of the analyst discover whenever the patient becomes more accessible, his defenses yield, and free-floating anxieties can be analyzed.

At the other end of the scale we meet the cycloid patient whose instability is manifested in mood swings and a tendency to act out. He may petulantly insist on daily interviews which he is compelled largely to waste by monotonous complaints, throwing the responsibility for the treatment in the lap of the analyst in whom he sees mainly the magic helper. This demonstrative dependency does not yet establish a profitable working relationship. In the system of defenses of the cycloid patient the erotization of anxiety stands out and may mislead the analyst. Only to the degree that these defenses can be melted, do anxiety and libido become available for the analytic work. A change of frequency sometimes brings frustration and infantile conflicts into focus, which the patient covered by petulance or pacified with daily interviews. A patient of this kind told me after a reduction of hours: "For the first time I have understood my dependency needs on you not with my head, but with my heart." Simultaneously a dream brought a lost memory of a terrifying desertion experience in the third year of her childhood, a tonsillectomy in which the parents failed her. The anxiety was relived in full force.

I have mentioned the schizoid and the cycloid types of patient. Mostly we are confronted with mixed types, as we meet various degrees of mixture between hysteric and obsessional symptomatology. A differentiation of frequency seems to me particularly to be recommended in chronic cases, character neuroses, where factors of arrested development outweigh the incidents of acute regressions. A neurosis with acute symptomatology, I think, needs daily, or near to daily, interviews as long as the pressure of actualized conflicts mobilizes anxieties. But when the patient has reached a higher degree of integration and self-sufficiency, he is highly encouraged by a reduction of sessions which acknowledges his progress. Once he has developed, besides the transference, a reliable realistic relation to the analyst, he can maintain the continuity of the work over even longer interruptions.

I have pointed out this variety of possibilities in order to warn against an inflexible ruling in matters of frequency. We have recently observed in the pediatric discipline a change from a rigidly instituted feeding schedule according to the clock to a demand schedule which arranges the frequency of feedings according to the needs of the infant. This change helps to establish a better rapport between mother and infant. It replaces the letter of the law by the spirit of mutual understanding. With the growing development of psychoanalysis we become able to learn from our pediatric colleagues to adapt ourselves better to the needs of our patients. I do not mean merely the consciously expressed needs, since these may at times be pathologically overheated demands which distort the deeper repressed real needs. We are of course interested in maintaining the regularity of our schedule. But when in addition to the natural tendency toward automatization of habits we press the institutionalization of a frequency rule—four weekly hours are analysis, three hours are not—then we regress from the spirit of psychoanalysis to a legalized form of it.

It is true, more inconvenience is implied when in matters of frequency we try to observe the needs of the patients in different phases of their analysis. But all technical rules, far from being unessential, are important observation points for manifestations of resistance, transference as well as countertransference. If we do not take an instituted frequency rule for granted, we have to come to terms with a possible unconscious aversion to seeing the patient more frequently, or with an unobserved hesitation to offer him more independence. Such investigation of our countertransference gives us an opportunity to become conscious of those factors in our own psychology which make us deviate from the benevolent neutrality which is the most effective attitude toward the patient and the therapeutic task. The factors of narcissistic counterresistance can be sorted out. After that, the countertransference reactions inform us about the patient's unconscious needs in a given situation. Glover called this daily self-scrutiny, which is of course not communicated to the patient, "the toilet of the analyst."

We can improve our technique when we use the analytic microscope in the mutual assessment of our work, when we dare to expose not only transference but also countertransference resistances in our analytic reports to each other. It is evident that detailed and intimate reports are only possible in smaller groups, for instance in a mutual consultation service such as Oberndorf has recommended in protracted, stagnating analyses. Such a more intimate exchange will make a streamlined ruling for mass consumption superfluous. It will strengthen the autonomy and spontaneity in our group work, while fixation of rules is a danger for a science that has set liberation from compulsion as an essential goal.

Let me sum up: The progress of psychoanalytic art and science depends to a high degree on the flexibility of psychoanalytic technique. In order to maintain our alertness to the essential analytic tasks of elucidating and dissolving resistance, transference and countertransference, we must avoid the dangers of habit formation, magic ceremonials, submission or rebellion in relation to rigid rules which do not correspond to the genuine needs of the patients. Deepened self-scrutiny of countertransference and intensified collaboration of psychoanalysts in mutual exchange will remove resistances of distrust and compulsion and maintain the freedom of spontaneous growth and creative development of psychoanalytic technique.

19

CARL A. WHITAKER

The Commitment to Intimacy

Once a therapist has accepted a patient for treatment, there are certain ethical responsibilities which are implicit, as well as certain legal responsibilities which are many times explicit. Recent literature has emphasized the manipulative aspects of psychotherapy and although the tactical and strategic phases are certainly significant and must be developed to the point where they are an aid in the patient's recovery, I believe that there must be more than a game pattern for the psychotherapy to be anything except a method for relieving symptoms. If the therapist believes in helping the patient expand his living and deepen it, the relationship itself must be deeper than a game.

I can decide to see a patient. I can decide to not commit myself to that patient for more than a game about his symptoms and a game about my function as a therapist. When therapy goes beyond the game-stage, the clarity of control is not automatic. I can not decide to commit myself to the patient on a preplanned basis; although once having committed myself, I can, within limits, decide the pattern of that commitment. However, this deciding is usually based on denial of response, rather than the choice of response. Beyond the decision to play the game, the therapist commits himself with the danger of uncontrolled involvement. Commitment implies a future time and is not merely a present state. The therapist plunging into the relationship presumes a decision that the end point of this

Reprinted with permission of the publisher from *Existential Psychiatry*, 1967, Vol. 6, 23.

relationship will be tolerable for him. Such a commitment has certain similarities to becoming pregnant. It may be possible to interrupt it, but this is a difficult and sometimes dangerous thing to do. However, to allow it to continue may, and frequently does, involve a lifetime of responsibility, with the constant challenge of being vulnerable to that person.

The object of committing oneself to intimacy with a patient is to obtain a heightened consciousness of oneself as a way of responding to crisis. Psychotherapy is an endless crisis, a rhythmic crisis of surge and ebb–a surge of intimacy, and the ebb of loneliness. Anxiety is part of the surge to intimacy just as despair is part of the ebb to loneliness. Yet, it is only by committing oneself to this rhythmic surge and ebb that one attains a state of aloneness, which is not loneliness (interpersonal isolation).

As each new patient-hour arrives, it's my own inner life that is at issue. Will I look at him and see an insignificant other, or, like the optical illusion, will I look at him and see my very self? Will I manage to be more and more naked with this other of myselves? Can I use him to be more with myself? Will he hurt me? Of course. Will I hurt him? I hope so. Can he take it when I hurt him? Yes, if I enjoy it. Can I make this a time when my significance to myself is increased one more quantum? Can I keep from hiding the impulse to lead his move to openness by one of my own? Can I expose my aloneness? Can I be available to an "other?"

Such commitment necessitates certain prerequisites. The therapist must first win the battle for structure. He must have been clear that this was his therapeutic process and that he is in charge of it. This is not just a meeting of two strangers. This is a meeting in which one person carries responsibility for the "unknowing" process, its timing and the reality factors in it. The therapist must win the battle for initiative or for joint beingness; that is, the therapist must force the patient to be and not act the patient role. This can only be done if the therapist insists on not being subject or object. He must insist on being himself and in his most intimate way. Endlessly asking himself in front of all who care to listen; Where am I? How am I? Is my inner self being or waiting? Being or doing? Being or refusing to be? Can I dare to share my inner self with me? Can I dare to be more full of myself? Each crisis is the effort to force myself to a greater commitment to intimacy with myself. From that, and only from that, can the patient get encouraged to be; that is, to commit himself further to intimacy with his person.

If I can commit myself to greater intimacy with myself, the patient will in his reciprocal aloneness be pressured to commit himself to a self-intimacy which is, in itself, authentic.

20

ELIZABETH E. MINTZ

On the Rationale of Touch in Psychotherapy

It is a source of recurrent amazement to me that the dimension of physical contact between therapist and patient has been almost ignored in literature on psychotherapy. Most contributors, even when discussing the patient-therapist relationship in detail, appear completely unaware of the possibility of touch as part of this relationship, or, like Menninger (1958, p. 40) regard any physical contact as "incompetence or criminal ruthlessness" on the part of the analyst.

Among contemporary experiential writers, physical contact is not anathematized, but is usually regarded as a way of expressing the concern or the emotional availability of the therapist (Gendlin, 1964, p. 145). What is typically absent is any extended consideration of the occasions on which physical contact may be therapeutically valuable, and when it may be counterindicated.[1]

Elsewhere (1969) I have discussed the historical background against which physical contact between analyst and patient became a tabu and have attempted to clarify whether touch is necessarily always contrary to the basic goals and methods of psychoanalysis, as distinct from psychotherapy in its broader sense. It was maintained that physical contact involving either the promise or the actuality of

1. An exception, striking because found in the work of so traditional an analyst as Edward Glover (1955, pp. 24-5), is a discussion of whether to shake hands, in which the point is made that this decision cannot be made as a general policy but only in terms of the patient's specific needs. He adds, "When in doubt behave naturally."

direct genital fulfillment is invariably inappropriate, primarily because the essential nature of therapy involves an encounter between a person who seeks to help and a person who seeks to be helped, a relationship which seems incompatible with the full mutuality of a healthy sexual relationship. It was, however, maintained that physical contact can be therapeutically appropriate in certain specific situations: As symbolic mothering at times when a patient cannot communicate verbally; to convey the therapist's acceptance at times when the patient is overwhelmed by self-loathing; and to strengthen or restore the patient's contact with the external world when it is threatened by anxiety. And it was further maintained that these situations are not confined to the treatment of overt or borderline psychotics, but can occur in deep analysis with patients who may possess considerable ego-strength.

We should explore further various aspects of touch as a part of therapeutic communication.

Touch as a natural part of a warm, ongoing relationship. In our society many people, though not all, find it natural to express warmth through occasional physical contact—a particularly friendly handshake, a touch on the shoulder when another person is depressed, an embrace of congratulations on being told of some success or happiness. Although many psychoanalysts are willing to admit confidentially that they do allow themselves such demonstrations with patients, they are in general considered inappropriate in the psychoanalytic relationship, in the belief that they may contaminate the transference and indeed may block the development of its negative aspects altogether.

I have conducted many analyses that, after the negative transference has worked through, were marked by deep feelings of mutual warmth, but in which there was never any overt physical contact except for an occasional handshake after a vacation. When contact seems natural, however, the question may be asked as to whether the transference may not be more contaminated by its avoidance than by its presence. The traditional viewpoint is that any bodily contact would serve as an artificial stimulant for fantasies that either the Oedipal wishes or the dependent infantile wishes might actually be gratified, that it would hinder the pure development of transference based on early object-relationships and introjects, and that it might block the development and expression of hostile feelings. Perhaps it might equally well be conjectured that a strict avoidance of physical contact under all circumstances could well repeat a physical rejection by the parents undergone by the patient as a child; could reinforce the denial of the physical aspect of human existence that is particularly characteristic of the obsessional and schizoid personalities in our culture and could increase the likelihood that patients, especially the two latter groups, might depersonalize the psychoanalytic relationship as a defense against experiencing feeling. Under such circumstance it would seem worthwhile for the analyst to consider whether his compliance with the traditional taboo against touch may not be serving the resistance.

Touch as gratification of the patient's infantile needs. If physical contact implies a danger of gratifying the patient to the point of interfering with his motivation toward growth and independence, the maintenance of touch as a taboo would indeed be appropriate. However, as has been pointed out even within the framework of the classical psychoanalytic structure (Roland, 1967), there are many patients, particularly those with severe neurotic character disturbances, who require a "real reparative object relationship" with the analyst, in addition to an opportunity to reproject and analyze harmful internalized objects. As such patients become increasingly able to seek and experience feelings, they often communicate a longing for the kind of nourishing and affectionate relationship absent in their childhoods; a relationship that in many cases can be gratified through words or other symbols, but that in the case of very immature personalities or very rigid and compulsive personalities may be most effectively expressed by the therapist's holding the patient.

Thus far, in my private practice with neurotics and well-compensated schizophrenics I have never found it appropriate to offer a patient the experience of being held in an individual session, although other therapists report having done so successfully with psychotic patients (Sechehaye, 1951). Whether the risks are realistic or whether they are based on the therapist's unresolved anxieties, risks do seem to exist of precipitating a massive intractable dependent transference or of eliciting intense hostility when the dependent needs cannot be subsequently satisfied on a mother-baby level or of evoking early incestuous fantasies before the patient is prepared to deal with them.

In groups, however, and especially in time-extended marathon groups,[2] the writer frequently has offered a participant the experience of being closely embraced for some time, perhaps for even fifteen minutes duration, by a parent-figure—usually by myself as a mother symbol, but sometimes by another woman who can serve as a

2. Here the term *marathon* refers to two-day intensive groups that focus on the individual needs of a limited number of participants, in contrast to larger "encounter groups" that have a different purpose and other values. It is my opinion (1967) that the former type of group may legitimately be regarded as an extension of the psychoanalytic situation.

mother symbol in the group, and sometimes by a male colleague or a male participant as a father figure.

This experience has not yet resulted in the clinging infantile dependency that is generally feared by responsible therapists. After being held, the participant almost invariably moves toward a deeper and more mature involvement with the group as a whole, offering help and support to others, or showing increased interest in his own reality problems.[3]

Touch as gratification of the patient's manipulative needs. The distinction between this meaning of touch, and the meaning discussed above, is sometimes difficult to make in practice, but is theoretically clear. There is a sharp distinction between the patient who reaches out for a temporary dependent and affectionate relationship that he was denied in childhood, and the patient who seeks to use contact as a way to control the therapist and avoid self-confrontation.

> A young man, a charmer of women who had always used his personal attractiveness to avoid responsibility, entered treatment in the depths of a depression, having worked with me some years previously in a different professional setting. At the end of a session in which he appeared genuinely despairing, he said, "You are my only hope," and turned at the door to embrace me. I accepted his embrace with a maternal feeling. No sexualization of the transference resulted, but it was my belated impression that the subsequent course of treatment, which on the whole was unsatisfactory, was adversely affected by my failure to recognize and analyze his gesture as an attempt to cajole me into ignoring the dependency and rage behind his depression.

> A young married woman, suffering from vague anxieties and a poorly-developed sense of identity originating in a childhood during which she had been treated as a pretty toy without feelings or needs of her own, said wistfully to me, "If only you would hold me—my mother never held me." Subsequently she had a dream that apparently was about a homosexual relationship with the analyst. She was offered no gesture of affection, nor was the dream analyzed as genuinely homosexual, but instead we discussed her effort to induce the analyst to treat her as a toy object, repeating her childhood experiences. Results of analysis were gratifying; the marital relationship became more mature and the patient developed a strong, sustained interest in socially worthwhile activity.

3. I have conducted 55 marathon groups, in which there have been perhaps 100 experiences of being held. Since the fear of precipitating infantile dependency is justifiably regarded as important in considering the maintenance of the tabu against touch in psychotherapy, it appears relevant to add that none of the participants in these groups whom I have held have sought a continuation of a personal or therapeutic relationship with me, with one exception. The exception was a young woman who had been referred for a marathon by a male colleague who hoped that she would decide to complete her analysis with a female analyst. She entered treatment with me, without indications of exaggerated dependency reactions.

These two cases fit into my tentative conjecture that when a patient is able to ask assertively for physical contact with the therapist, he is probably strong enough to be able to find it in nonsymbolic relationships outside therapy and may indeed be attempting to cajole or seduce the therapist. The patient who is genuinely in need of reparative physical contact is likely to be unable to express his need clearly.

Touch as a means of eliciting feelings about aggression. Physical expression of hostility purely as a catharsis in the therapeutic situation is of slight value in itself. However, such expression is often valuable as an aid in developing insight and in furthering the breakthrough of repressed feelings.

Here, as in the procedure of holding a patient, usually I confine physical expression of hostility to marathon groups. When a participant is struggling with hostile feelings toward the mother, the therapist may offer herself as a target or opponent. When hostility or competitiveness is experienced toward a father, or toward a peer, an appropriate male participant almost invariably volunteers to play the part of father surrogate. For these purposes, a variety of techniques can be used, including arm wrestling, which permit a satisfying expenditure of physical energy without damage to either participant or surroundings.[4]

> In a marathon group composed of colleagues, a competent mature, and well-defended man was telling his lifelong difficulty about expressing hostility toward his mother. I asked him to close his eyes, pretend that she was his mother, and grip her forearm as hard as possible (a procedure that can be easily sustained with very slight discomfort). With this physical expression of feeling to assist him, the participant was able to fantasy that he was actually speaking to his mother, and to express his bitterness and sense of deprivation, followed by a feeling of great relief. The participant subsequently spoke of this experience as an important breakthrough, and no awkwardness followed in his professional or social relationship with the writer.

Touch as an expression of the therapists' feelings. There seems no special reason to maintain that the therapist's expression of feeling is necessarily therapeutic only because it is genuine. However, the converse does appear to be true: Especially because many patients have been traumatized by constant uncertainty regarding the real feelings of their parents, any false gesture of acceptance or affection from the therapist could well be destructive, repeating the earlier trauma and diminishing the patient's confidence in his reality-testing.

4. I am indebted to Dr. William Schutze for introducing me to most of these techniques.

Use of physical contact, then, seems to require not only an understanding of the patient's psychodynamics and an awareness of the probable effects of touch at that moment, but also a readiness for touch on the part of the therapist. This may at first seem to place an unrealistic burden on the therapist, and certainly any therapist to whom this type of communication seems alien or improper should confine himself to verbal communication. However, these criteria for the use of touch are not really very different from the criteria for other types of therapeutic intervention, which also require understanding of the patient, a reasonably confident anticipation of the effect of the therapist's activity, and a reasonable degree of personal ease and comfort in the therapist.

The anxiety is sometimes expressed that any kind of physical contact may lead to inappropriate and destructive sexual acting-out. This argument seems specious: A therapist who could be swept away by touching a patient's hand or embracing a regressed patient could probably in any case not withstand the sustained intimacy of the therapeutic relationship.

If physical contact is to be another dimension of communication in therapy, it is probably important for the therapist to engage in continued self-training. He may, for example, frequently think back over a session, checking himself not only on his theoretical rationale but on the personal feelings that may have been involved in his communication, inasmuch as it is usually impossible to consider these questions fully in the immediate pressure of the session. Yet, again, this procedure is essentially no different from what the responsible therapist does with regard to verbal intervention. The term tabu[5] implies a prohibition that is maintained on the basis of tradition rather than rationality; to the extent to which physical contact in therapy is a tabu, there can be no place for it in what is hopefully a growing science.

5. This term was first suggested in regard to therapeutic touch by Ruth C. Cohn.

REFERENCES

1. Gendlin, E. T. "A Theory of Personality Change," in *Personality Change*, P. Worchel & D. Byrne, eds. New York: John Wiley & Son, 1964.
2. Glover, E. *The Technique of Psychoanalysis*. New York: International Universities Press, 1955.
3. Menninger, K. *Theory of Psychoanalytic Technique*. New York: Basic Books, 1958.
4. Mintz, E. "Time-Extended Marathon Groups." *Psychotherapy: Theory: Research and Practice*. Vol. 4, #2, May, 1967.
   ——— Touch and the Psychoanalytic Tradition. *The Psychoanalytic Review*. In press.
5. Roland, A. "The Reality of the Psycho-analytic Relationship and Situation in the Handling of Transference-Resistance." *International Journal of Psychoanalysis*, Vol. 48, Part 4, 1967.
6. Sechehaye, M. A. *Symbolic Realization*. New York: International Universities Press, 1951.

21

ALTHEA J. HORNER

To Touch—Or Not To Touch

In the eighth issue of *Voices,* Dr. John Rosen disagreed with Drs. Grotjahn and Wells[1] about the therapist's role as a provider of gratification. In the same issue Dr. Jules Masserman[2] described the great public appeal of Greatrakes the Stroaker during the seventeenth century and related this to the current appeal of the chiropractor or the masseur, all of them providing, through touch, the gratification of the comforting mother.

In the findings of Harlow[3] and the innate need for contact comfort in the monkey can be extended to the human being, then we should not be surprised to find that this need may arise in the therapy situation. The issue of touch in psychotherapy is—I am tempted to say, redundantly—a touchy one. Is there a place for "stroaking" in psychotherapy? Or should such gratification of need be withheld lest it hold out false promise for more, as Drs. Grotjahn and Wells suggest?

The John Rosens notwithstanding, physical contact between therapist and patient is generally frowned upon. These limits in therapy are supposedly set up to prevent sticky transference problems. There is no doubt that they also serve to prevent sticky countertransference problems as well.

Reprinted with permission of the author and publisher from *Voices*, 1968, Vol. 14, No. 2, 26-28.

1. Grotjahn, M. and Wells, P.H.: "Schizophrenogenic Trends in Therapy," *Voices*, Vol. 3, No. 2, 1967, 14-17.
2. Masserman, J.: "Physical Contact," *Voices*, Vol. 3, No. 2, 1967, 97.
3. Benjamin, Lorna S.: "Harlow's Facts on Affects," *Voices*, Vol. 4, No. 1, 1968.

But are there not times when contact comfort might serve not only to make the patient feel better at the moment, but also as a corrective emotional experience?

I will use myself as a clinical example of how the strict holding to these limits by the therapist may act to reinforce earlier negative experiences and self-perceptions.

I was born to a mother who could be tender and demonstrative towards the helpless baby, but who withdrew love when the child's developing will led to the first "no." Driven by a strong need for autonomy, I sacrificed maternal affection at an early age. I do not remember the last time I was held affectionately in my mother's arms. I grew up convinced that she did not love me, and questioned my lovability. Then I married a kind but undemonstrative man who grew up in a home where open affection was not shown. My need for touch, for "stroaking," for contact comfort, was once again thwarted. My self-image became more and more one of "untouchableness."

As a graduate student I went into psychotherapy where, from time to time, I would express my longing to have the therapist hold me. Each time I was told that my problem was that I wanted gratification instead of therapy. Now I had learned something new about myself. Not only was I untouchable, but my wish for comfort was "bad."

A few years later, facing a personal crisis, I had occasion to see another therapist for a short time. Undoubtedly in order to protect myself from being rebuffed once more, I told him at the start about my previous experience and wondered what he would do were I to express such a wish. He shared openly with me his feelings of anxiety at the prospect. I smiled and reassured him that this would not happen. But now I had learned still more about myself. I made people uncomfortable. My wish for contact comfort was frightening to others. It might drive them away from me. I was now not only untouchable and bad; I was also a danger to others.

I must also state here that, on the whole, both therapy experiences were enormously helpful, but a small pocket of iatrogenic pathology superimposed upon the original, was still with me.

Not too long ago I spent a week at the Esalen Institute at Big Sur, California, attending a workshop led by Dr. Herbert Otto on how to realize one's human potential, and another led by Virginia Satir on family therapy. Part of Dr. Otto's technique is the issuing of lapel buttons which indicate the individual's willingness to be touched. Suddenly I found myself in a situation in which touch was neither bad nor feared, but valued and encouraged.

Tentative at the start, but at the very end crying as another woman held me close, the whole structure of my negative self-image came crashing down. Once more, in Mrs. Satir's workshop during a marathon psychodrama, I found myself being held as a child by its mother when, sensing my anguish, she sat down on the floor beside me and gently held me in her arms. Men–women–it made no difference. The need for the kind of contact that says you are not untouchable, bad, or dangerous has no sex.

It is now almost a year later, and the process of change within me which started at Esalen has continued and gradually been integrated. And, not so surprisingly, my inner transformation has affected my approach to others. Being less guilty and anxious over taking the initiative in an encounter, I could allow myself greater openness and spontaneity. I took greater risks but then I also reaped greater rewards. For equally predictable, the response of others to me was also changed, including that of my husband and my patients.

One might very correctly argue that the Esalen experience was not psychotherapy. This is true–at least, not officially. But I find myself wondering now–why not? Why can't this kind of experience take place in the private encounter between therapist and patient? I'm a little afraid of it myself because I am aware of the danger that a therapist like myself might use the relationahip for self gratification . . . which brings me around full circle. Drs. Grotjahn and Wells tell me it is bad technique. I will be a danger to the patient. And so I find myself wondering about the experiences of other therapists. What do most therapists do when the patient's need for contact comfort becomes a here-and-now issue?

22

HENDRIK M. RUITENBEEK

Freud As Therapist: Include The Patient In Your World

I said on leaving that it would be good if all psychoanalysts showed his (Freud) open-mindedness and good sense. . . . "If they are my pupils, they do," said Freud.
–from *Fragments of an Analysis with Freud* by Joseph Wortis

We all know by now that Freud never intended to create an impersonal and detached analyst. For those who have read in Jones' biography of Freud and elsewhere[1] about the contacts Freud had and maintained with his patients, it seems clear that Freud himself was far from detached or cold in his contacts with patients. Unfortunately we have only rather meager documentation about the interaction between Freud and his patients,[2] but Kaplan notes that[3]

1. To cite a few works that have some material on Freud's contacts with patients: Franz Alexander, Samuel Eisenstein, and Martin Grotjahn, eds., *Psychoanalytic Pioneers* (New York: Basic Books, 1966). Martin Freud, *Sigmund Freud: Man and Father* (New York: The Vanguard Press, 1958). Joseph Wortis, *Fragments of an Analysis with Freud* (New York: Bobbs-Merrill Co., 1954). (One of the very few personal accounts of an analysis with Freud). Vincent Brome, *Freud and His Early Circle*, (New York: Morrow, 1968). H. F. Peters, *My Sister, My Spouse* (New York, Norton, 1962). Rudolph Binion, *Frau Lou* (Princeton: Princeton University Press, 1968).

2. Since many of Freud's patients are still alive, any documentation must be postponed for at least another generation. Nevertheless, some of Freud's patients have shared their experience with the public. Hilda Doolittle (the poet, H. D.) wrote a touching account of her analysis with Freud. See *Tribute to Freud* by H. D. (New York: Pantheon, 1956). Unfortunately she is one of the very few who has been willing to discuss her work with Freud.

3. Donald M. Kaplan, "Freud and his own Patients," *Harper's Magazine*, December 1967, p. 99.

"Naturally Freud's character—his almost naive earnestness—found expression in his daily clinical practice, in his actual conduct with patients. In his therapeutic activities, which flash with character, there are awesome glimpses of his great purpose that have remained comparatively neglected in the dissemination of his thought." We can also certainly form something of an opinion about Freud's approach to his patients by consulting other available sources. Through her own reports[4] and her eminent biographers,[5] Lou Andreas-Salome, for example, one of Freud's most esteemed and intimate pupils, presents us with a picture of Freud that confirms his warmth, his attachments and his *own* awareness of his mistakes and/or shortcomings.[6]

Few analysts, if any, have written about their desire to incorporate their awareness of error into their clinical worlds. Much has been published on countertransference, but little that deals with the social and cultural context of the analyst's world.[7]

Admittedly, the analyst's is not the world he presents to his patient; at most, he presents a small part of that world. Patient's questions about *his* interests, *his* politics, *his* feelings about life in general, have all too often been answered (when they have been answered) in terms of the patient's motivations for questioning the analyst. True enough, reticence and this challenging approach of the analyst have often led the patient to produce important material, which in turn contributes to the process of analysis.

4. See *Mein Dank an Freud* (Wein; Internationaler Psychoanalytischer Verlag, 1931); Ernst Pfeiffer, ed., *Lebensruckblick* (Zurich; Max Niehans, 1951); Ernst Pfeiffer, ed., *In der Schule Bei Freud* (Zurich; Max Niehans, 1958). Also English translation, *The Freud Journal of Lou Andreas-Salome* (New York: Basic Books, 1964).

5. H. F. Peters, *op. cit.*; Rudolph Binion, *Frau Lou* (Princeton; Princeton University Press, 1968).

6. Joan Riviere gives a very vivid account of her analysis with Freud in an article, "An Intimate Impression," *The Lancet*, Sept. 20, 1939, p. 765, where she writes "Like his psychology, his personality was really one to concern itself with individuals. The aloofness, which was never indeed coldness or hauteur, but rather indifference to superficialities, vanished, and one met a vivid, eager mind seizing on every detail with astonishing interest and attention. . . .My first analytic hour with him he opened—contrary to rule and inadvisably—saying, 'Well, I know something about you already; you had a father and a mother!' " Jones writes about Freud's indiscretion in remarking, "When James Strachey went to study with Freud I wrote a letter of introduction, not entirely complimentary, telling Freud what little I knew of him at that time. In an early session Freud went into the next room, fetched the letter and read it aloud to him". (Ernest Jones, *The Life and Work of Sigmund Freud*, Vol. II, p. 410).

7. The publication *Voices* of the American Academy of Psychotherapists has been very courageous in publishing various accounts of therapists about their feelings on patients.

It should be noted, nevertheless, that the patient who totally reveals himself to the analyst, might take comfort in knowing his analyst in other ways than on the strictly analytic level.

Existential analysts, such as Ronald Laing,[8] have advocated the dialogue[9] as an analytic device for rousing the patient. In such an analytic situation, the dialogue will have to include *feelings* and even opinions of the analyst. Dialogue cannot be restricted if it is to work. To be effective in the psychotherapeutic process it must be open and free. The analyst who is warm, concerned, frank and open, cannot but express some of his own feelings about what the patient brings up in the analytic situation. The commitment of the analyst to the world in terms of political, social, and cultural questions cannot but be converged to the patient. Patients have opinions, but so do analysts. Freud never shrank from expressing his opinions about people and issues in a very frank manner to his analysands.[9]

Freud's pupils were similarly forthright. Those who have read the notebooks of Anais Nin know how open and committed Rank was in the analytic situation as he related to Miss Nin: I do not believe in long drawn out psychoanalysis. I do not believe in spending too much time exploring the past, delving into it. I believe neurosis is like a virulent abscess, or infection. It has to be attacked powerfully in the present. Of course, the origin of the illness may be in the past, but the virulent crisis must be dynamically tackled."[10]

Nothing is more discouraging to a patient than inability to recognize his analyst as a human being. No analyst should be only a talking robot repeating stock phrases and using them as a means of keeping patients completely at arms length. Even strict Freudian analysis should remain a fully human affair.

Well-balanced and well-analyzed therapists are *able, capable,* and *willing* to share their own feelings with the patient. These feelings do not necessarily have to be profound. A remark about some event on the political or social scene, a comment on a movie being mentioned, perhaps some observation on the death of a famous person, a reaction to a strike, a casual remark about travel plans, even, on occasion, taking notice of a shared liking for some food—all of this

8. See especially his *The Divided Self* (London: Tavistock, 1959) and *The Politics of Experience* (New York: Pantheon, 1967). (Thomas Szasz, too has advocated use of dialogue in the therapeutic process. See *Ethics of Psychoanalysis*, New York: Basic Books, 1965).

9. Jones in Chapter 16, Volume II of his *Freud* cites some telling material about Freud's relationship with his analysands. Wortis, *op. cit.*, has very interesting observations about Freud's approach to his analysands.

10. *The Diary of Anais Nin,* Vol. 1 (New York: Harcourt, Brace & World 1966), p. 277.

creates an atmosphere in which patient and analyst experience mutual trust.

We have entered a stage in the contemporary analytic situation where age-old (fifty years old really!) *taboos* are likely to be dismissed with or at least to be seriously questioned. Elizabeth Mintz' article on touch and the psychoanalytic tradition (Chapter 21) and some other recent papers on this subject[11] indicate a change in attitude toward significant bans such as that on touch in the psychoanalytic situation.

Part of all this is that we have been burdened with a *pseudo* heritage of the first generation of psychoanalysts. I maintain that the distortions of the second generation of analysts about their teachers' concepts and opinions is simply staggering. The early analysts were on the whole informal (regardless of their formal background) in their approach to the psychoanalytic situation. They were warm and open; the German term *gemütlich* connotes such a climate, something that American analysts find difficult to achieve (probably because of cultural reasons).[12] I have always had the impression that many traditional analysts were rather rigid about their interaction with patients. It can be said that too often we see our patients as patients and not persons. Hence we tend to forget Freud's remarks about psychoanalysis *not* being a part of medicine,[13] which has implications for the psychoanalytic situation going far beyond the limited issue of lay analysis.

Freud regarded psychoanalysis as an independent discipline, and he often expressed the desire to see psychoanalysis clarified as a branch of the humanities. Some of his most outstanding pupils were lay analysts. Otto Rank considered himself an artist; Hans Sachs was trained in law before entering psychoanalysis. Lou Andreas-Salome was a writer of note before she became a pupil of Freud. Too often we forget that psychoanalysis is a gift (as Lou Andreas-Salome termed it) or a talent.

None of this implies that we should abandon the traditional psychoanalytic situation. Patients still will have to be on time, not break their appointments, and pay their fees. But within that struc-

11. See especially *Voices*, Summer, 1968, the entire issue is devoted to acting out.

12. I have come to doubt the so-called openness of Americans *per se* and now believe that there is far more rigidity in the American personality than they would like to admit. And this character trait certainly does not make flexible and relaxed analysts.

13. See his book *The Question of Lay-Analysis*, Standard Edition, Vol. XX, which has been ignored by the psychoanalytic establishment but contains some gems on the general state of psychoanalysis.

ture there is much more leeway for interaction between analyst and patient than many analysts have realized until now.

Why should the patient not see his analyst as the person he really is? Why deny that analysts have their likes and dislikes, too? The analyst all too often employs clever evasions as a technique that allows him to escape from a serious and genuine question by a patient? The analyst can show his patients his world (and likes and dislikes) by various means. Freud liked Greek and Egyptian antique sculpture and kept it around his office. From the pictures we have of that room one would hardly think of an analyst's office at all.

As a matter of fact, Martin Freud describes how his father kept a favorite dog in his consulting room during the sessions.[14]

> Jofi was father's favorite and never left him, not even when he treated patients. Then he would lie motionless near his desk, that desk adorned with its Greek and Egyptian antique statuettes, while he concentrated on the treatment of patients. He always claimed . . . that he never had to look at his watch to decide when the hour's treatment should end. When Jofi got up and yawned, he knew the hour was up; she was never late in announcing the end of a session, although father did admit that she was capable of an error of perhaps a minute, at the expense of the patient. Freud did not hesitate to share in effect that what he cherished in life with his patients.

Another example of Freud's relaxation with his patients appears in Hilda Doolittle's little book.[15] She relates that before her analytic hour she always ran into a charming, impressive man and apparently Freud volunteered the following information on him:

> . . . The Professor was 77 at the time of our first sessions. I was 47. Dr. van der Leeuw [the man she met] was considerably younger. He was known among them, the Professor told me, as the Flying Dutchman. He was an eminent scholar. He had come officially to study with the Professor with the idea of the application of the principles of psychoanalysis to general education. . .[16]

Many contemporary analysts would find it improper, to say the least, to discuss one patient with another in this fashion. But one gets the impression that the ground rules in Vienna were not so strict as they are and have been in New York. The coldness and the impersonal atmosphere of some contemporary analysts' consulting rooms reflect their often rather rigid and inflexible attitude towards their patients.

We must realize that our world is also our patients' world. We demand that the patient put himself on the line; we ask for his complete commitment to the process of psychoanalysis. We require

14. Martin Freud, *op. cit.*, pp. 190-191.
15. H. D., *op. cit.*.
16. *op. cit.*, p. 4.

him to open up his world for us, a painful and trying experience. More of us should recognize that the trust we seek in the psychoanalytic situation can only be established when we, too, open up and reveal ourselves. And this not for our own purposes but solely for the patient's interest. The well-trained and insightful analyst is very well able to detect when the patient is trying to manipulate him. Nor will the analyst hesitate to communicate his discovery to the patient.

Far more than in Freud's time, our patients—alienated and lonely as they are—need to feel that the analyst is committed and concerned for them. After all, the age of repression is gone; now we encourage our patients to express themselves to the fullest in order that they, too, may discover their hidden talents. The effectiveness of the analyst depends to a large extent upon the character of his commitment to the patient. No contemporary analyst can evade the need to accept that commitment, nor can he escape from the obligation to establish a real and human relationship by repeating the cliches of an analytic orthodoxy which Freud himself disavowed.

23

JAMES F.T. BUGENTAL

Psychotherapy as a Source of the Therapist's Own Authenticity and Inauthenticity

One of the largely unexpected rewards and hazards of writing a book, I find, is the personal response it evokes from some readers. When *The Search for Authenticity*[1] was published several years ago, I had not anticipated that from time to time I would receive moving communications expressive of the responses of people who deeply heard what I sought to say and who gave me the gift of telling me about that hearing.

One such person, a young man who lived some distance away, wrote gratefully of the personal meaningfulness to him of having read my book. I responded, and we exchanged several letters. He wrote that he would be visiting Los Angeles and would like to meet me, so we set a time. When he came in, he indicated that he was thinking of moving to Los Angeles and would like to enter therapy with me. Then, 15 minutes after he entered the office, he was weeping—and he was weeping because he was so disappointed in me!

He was able to say how he experienced me as so much less authentic, so much less an embodiment of what I had written and what he had read, than he had expected. And, of course, he was right. I have wept bitterly myself for the same reason.

Apparently the young man who wept for me—and for himself, of course—was at one level weeping chiefly because he was again disappointed in his search for an ideal image figure with which to

Reprinted with permission of the author and publisher from *Voices*.

1. J. F. T. Bugental, *The Search for Authenticity: An Existential Analytic Approach to Psychotherapy*. (New York: Holt, Rinehart & Winston), 1965.

identify. However, it is also true that he correctly discerned my own inauthenticity.

The Demands of Reconstructive Therapy

I want to discuss, rather candidly, some of the influences operating on the therapist as a person which tend to increase or decrease his authenticity. My focus here is the relation between the therapist and his patient. I think we have been too hesitant in facing up to some of these matters and what they may mean for us as persons, for our patients, and for our relations with our surrounding society.

My concern is primarily with therapists who practice what, for lack of a better name, we can call long-term, intensive or reconstructive psychotherapy. This will include much of psychoanalysis, existential therapy, depth therapy, and so on. It will clearly not include behavior therapy, the various types of short term and ameliorative therapies, or what Wolberg[2] designates as reeducative therapies.

Probably the best way to characterize the kinds of therapy I am discussing is to say that they usually involve three or more contacts a week over several years, intimate and direct encounters between therapist and patient, and relatively little attention to the intercurrent life situation but relatively heavy concentration on the intrapsychic life. Quite possibly a key distinguishing characteristic is that the therapist has made this work his major life activity for some years. I believe that the impact on the therapist himself of many years of involvement with the deepest levels of the human experience is a uniquely formative one and one with products of which we know very little.

Another way to specify just what kind of psychotherapy I am interested in is to discuss therapeutic goals. I am thinking of a process which seeks to aid the patient in effecting fundamental changes in his life orientation. This is quite different from an effort to change undesirable habits, to overcome a trauma, or to resolve a conflict. To be sure, in order to deal with the habit, the trauma, or the conflict, it may turn out to be necessary to go behind them, so to speak, and to get at the life orientation which underlies them. When this is the case, then the therapeutic endeavor is of the order which I am attempting to characterize.

I want to discuss a therapy which seeks to change the life orientation of the person—that is, an existential therapy. I do not believe that such existential therapy has been adequately described; more-

2. L. R. Wolberg, *The Technique of Psychotherapy*, 2nd. ed., (New York: Grune and Stratton), 1967.

over, I do not believe it can be successfully carried out in many instances within the framework of our traditional and public conceptions of the therapist's and the patient's roles. Or to put the matter more affirmatively and more baldly: I think that in many instances, successful existential therapy requires the therapist to go beyond the usual conceptions of good taste,[3] accepted practice, professional ethics, and, I am tempted to add, common sense. Moreover, I would propose that at least some of these "goings beyond" are required by the very nature of the therapeutic task undertaken.

The central thesis I am advancing is that intensive psychotherapy requires the therapist continually to risk his own life stance, his own modes of being in the world. In the process he will find himself repeatedly involved with his patients in ways which are quite at variance with the traditional model of therapeutic detachment—ways which are much more to be seen as two human beings struggling for their lives rather than as a scientific doctor treating an appreciative patient. Finally, the failure of our professional community to recognize and accept this requirement of involved struggling leads to additional inauthenticity on the part of the therapist, with resulting cost to himself and those close to him, including his patients.

Therapy which is designed to produce genuine character change is a hazardous, unfairly demanding, socially borderline undertaking for both participants.

The Patient-Person and the Therapeutic Process

When Don Smith comes to me for psychotherapy, he comes because he finds that he is not content with his way of having his life, with his way of being in the world. Don wants to change some part of that way of being in the world. Perhaps he finds that he cannot really gain much satisfaction in his relations with other people. Perhaps he knows that he has seldom been able in what he does to work to what he feels is his true capacity. Again it may be that he has succeeded well in his work and has what seems to be a good marriage, yet he is haunted by a sense of meaninglessness or incompleteness in his life. Whatever the words which Don uses in talking with me, his complaint is a cry for help in rescuing his life from a drift or trend that Don finds inexorable and yet unacceptable in a degree which may range from annoying to terrorizing.

As an aside, we may note that it is likely that sooner or later we will discover that Don has a secret proviso in his plea for help—

3. See—as a prime instance—the courageous piece on "The Affair," by O. Spurgeon English, *Voices*, No. 10, Winter 1967.

sometimes secret from himself as well as withheld from me. This proviso says, "Help me change this or that part of my life, but leave undisturbed this other part, this special, this vital part of me." And, of course, experienced therapists well know that this is just exactly what cannot be done. Therapeutic doctrine is generally clear that the withheld secret part is very apt to be at, or very close to, the nucleus of the neurosis—or in more existential terms, to be integral to the main resistances[4] to authentic being in the world.

But let us think further about Don Smith and his seeking for help to change his way of being in the world. Just who or what is Don Smith? Who or what is it that wants to change his way of being in the world? The answer is ultimately that Don Smith is just this very way he has of being in the world! And just to make matters a bit more confusing, let us recognize that the exchanges between therapist and patient—between Don Smith and me—will be in terms of his way of being in the world. So now here indeed is a pretty state of things: Don Smith, as a way of being in the world, seeks to change Don Smith's way of being in the world, through using Don Smith's way of being in the world!

Were this the whole of the story, I think it would be manifest that genuine character therapy is an impossibility, an absurdity, a self-contradiction. However, many therapists and patients have seen empirically that such therapy *is* possible and that true basic changes can and do occur in some people in the therapeutic situation. Moreover, the introduction of the therapist does not constitute a valid resolution of the paradox, for it is also true that some people effect such fundamental changes without the aid of a psychotherapist. Thus, I think, we are provided with something approximating a critical experiment: Obviously if Don Smith is *only* his way of being in the world, he cannot change his way of being in the world solely by employing his way of being in the world. The dilemma is only to be resolved by recognizing that Don Smith is indeed his way of being in the world, but he is also something more.

I have suggested before[5] that we may be handicapped in our thinking about such problems as the above by our unthinking equation of the terms "person," "I," "me," and "self." I will not review here that discussion, but I want to pull out one aspect of it which is important for our purpose. I propose that we need to distinguish what may be termed the "I-process" from the "Self." By the *I-process* I will designate the existence which is the essence, the pure subjectivity, of the person. This, it seems to me, is not substantive,

4. Bugental, *op. cit.*
5. *Ibid.*

has no attributes, but is pure process. In an over-simplified fashion we may conceive of the *I-process* as a feeling of awareness or consciousness-and-choosing.

On the other hand, we may conceive of the *Self* as the sum of the awareness of the *I-process* about its own being. Thus the *Self* is purely object, is not aware, is substantive and attributive. Raimy,[6] one of the first to study the self empirically, defined it as "a learned perceptual system which functions as an object in the perceptual field of the behaver" (p. 331). The *Self*, then, is the way of being in the world. To confuse the *Self* and the *I-process* is equivalent, in this way of conceiving matters, to confusing the automobile and its driver. As someone observed, "Structure is the secretion of process." We may add, the *Self* is the secretion of the *I-process*.

Don Smith, the *I-process*, thus comes to psychotherapy for help in changing his *Self*, his way of being in the world. In the therapeutic course he will exercise his feelingful awareness and his choice-making potential to examine and modify his learned ways of being in the world. Thus our paradox is, at least heuristically, resolved.

Now let us take a look at the nature of that therapeutic course. In a very over-simplified fashion we may say that Don Smith must do three things: First, he must become more fully aware of just how he is in the world–that is, of the sort of *Self* he has developed over the years. In this process he will increasingly experience the points of his resistance to authenticity of being, the points which are the roots of his distress or dissatisfaction with his life. Second, if he is to effect any changes, he must become aware of his essential being as something somehow apart from any of the specifics of his *Self*. Finally, once he has emancipated his feelingful awareness, and, choosing from its constricting equation with his *Self*, he can then set about changing his way of being in the world.

The key step in the whole matter is the second one: Don Smith must discover that he is not just what he has always been or what he or others see him to be. Without this emancipation, Don can go on interminably in therapy, accumulating endless information about his *Self* resolving to do things differently and finding the futility of what Rollo May[7] calls the exercise of "Victorian will power." Yet this key step is the most difficult, the most threatening, the most resisted of all. This is so because it involves the confrontation and incorporation of existential anxiety.

6. V. C. Raimy, The Self-concept as a Factor in Counseling and Personality Organization. Unpublished doctoral dissertation (Columbus, Ohio: Ohio State University), 1943.

7. R. May, in R. B. MacLeod, ed., *The Unfinished Business of William James*. In press.

To clarify the nature of this anxiety, let us recognize that the *Self* arises as a way of getting about in the world as in the automobile-driver analogy above. The *Self* gives us a vehicle for meeting the (apparently) practical demands of daily life. In this way, the *Self* becomes the accumulated composite of our ways of meeting the anxiety that arises out of the very awareness of being. Paul Tillich[8] suggested that this existential anxiety takes three main forms: The anxiety of fate and death, the anxiety of guilt and condemnation, and the anxiety of emptiness and meaninglessness. To these I find it helpful to add two additional forms, the anxiety of pain and destruction and the anxiety of loneliness and isolation. How the forms of existential anxiety are classified, however, is of small importance. The significant matter is that Don Smith must endure letting go of the very ways he has built up throughout his life for coping with the existential anxiety *if* he is to free his *I-process* from his *Self* and thus make true characterological change possible. For Don Smith's character structure is, at root *his* ways of dealing with the fact and the anxiety of being.

This letting go of the *Self* is no small matter. It is fraught with the most extreme pain and terror. It is often accompanied by dreams, fantasies, and impulses toward insanity, suicide, and death. The patient accurately senses that his old *Self* is dying, that he is relinquishing the world (or at least his way of experiencing it). It is here that the withheld secret to which I referred earlier becomes the cruel ransom for a renewed life. The secret turns out to be the nuclear, inauthentic way in which the patient seeks to give substance to his being in the world. The parallels are numerous to the teachings of various religious systems: The injunctions to die in order to be reborn, the admonitions to forsake all else to follow the new teachings, the disclosure of the world of illusion that stands between the seeker and his goal.

The Therapist-Person and the Therapeutic Process

Now it is time to leave our focus on the patient and turn our attention to the therapist. What are his role and function, and what is the impact on him of carrying them out? Again, in simplified form, we can say that the therapist's task is to aid the patient in the exploration of his way of being in the world and in the recognition of those ways in which the patient is inauthentic in his confrontation of the existential conditions of his being and their attendant anxiety,

8. P. Tillich, *The Courage To Be*. (New Haven: Yale University Press), 1952. (Best chapter is 1.)

and to support the patient in his efforts to free his *I-process* from his *Self*. The central faculty through which the therapist does these things is his own inner awareness, his own confronting of the conditions of being and their anxious elements, and his own freeing of his subjective feelingful awareness from the constriction of any one way of being in the world.

But this is asking too much of most, if not all, of us therapists! We are not saints or gurus. We have our own needs for seeming security against the awful dread of seeing existence nakedly. We cannot dwell in this world as pure process. And so we compromise. *We accompany our patients as far as our own tolerance permits at any point with any given patient.* Sometimes we can risk more, sometimes less. Vaguely we recognize what the Buddhists have told us that all is illusion, that there is no right way of being in the world and that all ways are *ad hoc,* but we concentrate on that teaching's application to our patients and slide past its earthquaking significance for our own living. Frequently we see how the established, socially approved ways are the results of many men compromising together and thus are always in some measure less than satisfactory for any one given man. And, if we try to hold true, we dwell always in a borderland where the fixed certainties of other men become all too mutable, where the winds of existential anxiety repeatedly creep through the chinks in the walls of our defenses, and where—to more than redress the balance and yet to increase the threat—the challenge to further growth and emergence is always present.

Thus far, I've discussed these matters rather abstractly for the most part. I wanted to sketch in rather quickly what I feel to be the emotional setting in which the therapist works. I have done so in a rather dogmatic and summary fashion in order to set the issue somewhat starkly. Now let us consider the products of this state of affairs in the lives of therapists. As a starter, I think that the therapist needs by word and by implication to practice a deception (and often he will be deceiving himself as well): He must lead the patient to believe that he (the therapist) knows a safe route through the dangers of subjective basic encounter and major life change and that he will lead the patient along that safe road. Actually there is not—nor can there be—such a safe road. Both patient and therapist will, very literally, gamble with their lives. Unless patient and therapist are able to let go in some measure from the safe and the known, no deep change will occur. Moreover, there is no guarantee that they will "get back." Acting out, neurosis, psychosis, or other life disruption in the therapist are real possibilities. Such therapy as we are discussing is a phenomenon of a borderland between the reality-tested and the artistic, between psychosis and sanity, between the ethical and the unethical, between the socially accepted and the socially disruptive. The fearful intimacy of deep therapy can scarcely be overstated. It seems to me that psychotherapists have more than their "average share" of marital difficulties and divorces, more need to return to therapy for themselves, deeper bonds with like-minded therapists, more violations of social and ethical standards, more going beyond the usual bounds of what is thought of as acceptable practice.

The Breaking of Traditional Limits

What do I mean by going beyond accepted practice? Fortunately I can answer that question rather explicitly and anonymously, thus protecting the guilty and the courageous—who may well be the same people.

In 1962, I had the opportunity to administer a questionnaire on therapeutic practices to a group of 50 highly experienced psychotherapists representing the three major mental health professions. I asked them to say whether certain practices were conceivable under any conditions in their psychotherapeutic work. They were not asked to confess whether such instances had actually occurred. A sampling of the answers will illustrate my central thesis:

—Nearly 90 per cent accepted the idea of openly expressing their anger (this means more than simple annoyance or exasperation) at the patient.

—Almost 80 per cent might tell the patient about their own unresolved fears and anxieties.

—About 80 per cent accepted the possibility of issuing commands to a patient about something he should do in his extra-therapy life.

—About 75 per cent of them said it was conceivable that they might yell and shout at a patient.

—About 75 per cent could conceive of being in an embrace with a patient.

—Fully 75 per cent could accept encouraging the patient to role-play with them behaviors which had previously been avoided, such as hostile or seductive actions.

—Better than 70 per cent would under some circumstances go for a drink with a patient or socialize with him in either the patient's or the therapist's home.

—About 70 per cent might belittle, taunt, insult, or ridicule a patient.

—Around 70 per cent also might convey to a patient that the patient was in some way unique or special among the therapist's patients.

–About 70 per cent might share dreams or fantasies of their own with a patient.

–About 60 per cent might encourage a patient to break or damage office objects of minor monetary value.

–About 60 per cent admitted that a patient might be nude or nearly so during a session.

–Slightly over 50 per cent might engage in business transactions with the patient.

–About 50 per cent could conceive a situation in which the therapist sexually stimulated the patient or the reverse.

–About 40 per cent could conceive a situation in which they and a patient would remove some or all of their clothing during a session.

–But, interestingly, only about 25 per cent of the therapists could imagine loaning a patient money or asking sizable advance payments as a way of borrowing from him!

How representative this sample of therapists is, I do not know. They were drawn from all over the country and from widely varied training backgrounds and practicing situations. They were, for the most part, experienced and successful. All had had personal therapeutic experiences. I think it is likely that, while the percentages may not be statistically reliable, the general trend I am trying to depict is indeed present.

These examples suggest the experimentation that is going on. I shall have to use a more hearsay report to expand our recognition.

To my knowledge, as gained from patients and from other therapists, the following all have occurred with therapist's explicit or tacit approval, and at least nominally as a part of the therapy:

–A patient destroyed a rather expensive chair with his bare hands.

–A female patient frequently was nude and sometimes acted sexually provocatively. The therapist acknowledged his response, including showing that he had an erection.

–A male therapist and his female patient had sexual intercourse on a number of different occasions.

–Two men in a group fought until both were bloodied and exhausted.

–An entire therapy group, including the therapist, stripped and each person in turn embraced a woman who was leaving the group.

–A woman patient and a man patient wrestled angrily and quite seriously during a group session.

–An entire group held a husky man patient down while he struggled with all his strength to break loose.

–A therapy group regularly meets weekly, but once a month, they meet in the nude.

—A male patient exposed his female therapist's breasts and nursed on them.

Chiefly, of course, sexual and aggressive or hostile acts are involved. As Freud noted, these are the areas of our most severe conflicts. But often the underlying issues have to do with intimacy, conformity, courage to initiate, or dread of responsibility. Some years ago we would have dismissed the above instances as acting out or violations of accepted practice and thus of ethical codes. I propose that we can no longer so comfortably sweep them under the rug.

We are discovering that social and professional codes of behavior—while certainly useful in a mass society where people must, it seems, be treated as objects—may often serve as resistances to authentic being. Such codes may serve as "secrets" in the way I have characterized above and thus constrict the emancipation of the human potentials of patients and therapists alike.

Pressures Operating on the Therapist

I neither condemn nor approve any of these practices. Rather, I call for opening this entire matter to discussion so that we may aid each other in sorting out the authentic and the inauthentic in ourselves and in our practices.

Let me specualte on some of the forces which are acting on therapists. These forces powerfully affect therapists in all aspects of our being. Psychotherapy involves a therapist in:

—Intimacy, of a particular kind, greater than is possible in any other relation.

—Recognition that a two-way relationship is the only authentic relationship, i.e., rejection of one-way intimacy.

—Dealing in depth and detail with the most personal, the most revealing, the most socially forbidden aspects of our lives.

—Many hours devoted to this intimacy.

—Exposure in this intimate manner to a variety of personalities.[9]

—The tradition for the therapeutic work to be carried on in secret and seclusion. There can be little doubt that this kind of setting facilitates the necessarily intimate work of authentic exploration, but it also makes more likely inauthentic and acting-out possibilities and makes possible the experimental and unorthodox activities I have exemplified above.

9. Simply on a statistical basis the odds are great that sooner or later the therapist will encounter someone who matches him better emotionally and personally than any of the ordinarily-arrived-at-extra-therapeutic relations he may have.

–The self-selection, often largely on unconscious bases, through which professionals elect to channel a major portion of their work into the practice of this sort of psychotherapy as contrasted with the other avenues available to their talents. Almost certainly a high percentage of those of us who take this path have the need to find personal significance in the response of others, to express Messianic impulses, to grapple with what we feel are the fundamental issues of life, and to seek some degree of contending with existential anxiety through our patients.

–The impetus to constant growth and change in oneself which comes from working toward those goals with others who are courageously, frighteningly, but continuingly meeting their own anxieties with the therapist.

Conclusion

I have ranged rather widely to suggest a variety of influences which operate on the therapist who seeks to aid his patients at the most fundamental or existential levels. Perhaps I can summarize my thesis in the following manner: Any psychotherapy which seeks to aid the patient in changing his life orientation requires the employment of the most powerful force in the world: human relationship. Thus there is certain to be a problem of the therapist's involvement with his patients and of the effects of his work on his own life. That involvement and those effects are inevitable, appropriate, dangerous, healing, and may even be tragic. We are in the very early stages of learning to use that most powerful force which is the relationship of one person to another. It is beyond question that some will be hurt and that some hurts will be excessive. We can only seek ways to reduce such costs. We must not abandon the quest to learn to use that force.

We need more discussion of these issues, more honest presentation of them in our professional literature,[10] more acceptance of the inevitable costs with support for those hurt rather than a punitive reaction, and, finally, we need to reexamine our professional and social codes to make a place for the deeper realities about the human experience which our work is disclosing. Psychotherapists and their patients are social change agents, and they should accept this responsibility.

10. *Voices* has pioneered in the presentation of more candid and realistic material pertaining to the practice of psychotherapy, "saying it like it is."

Bibliography

Abraham, K. "First Prenatal Stage of the Libido," in *Selected Papers*. London: Hogarth, 1927, pp. 268-230.

________ *Collected Papers*. London: Hogarth, 1949.

Arieti, S. *Interpretation of Schizophrenia*. New York: Robert Brunner, 1955.

Balint, M. "Changing Therapeutic Aims and Techniques in Psychoanalysis," *Int. J. Psycho-Anal.*, Vol. 31, p. 117, 1950.

________ "The Three Areas of the Mind: Theoretical Considerations," *Int. J. Psycho-Anal.*, Vol. 39, p. 328, 1958.

Bebring, E. "The Mechanism of Depression, in P. Greenace, ed., *Affective Disorders*. New York: International Universities Press, 1953.

Beres, D. "Communication and the Creative Process," *J. Amer. Psychoanal. Assoc.*, Vol. 5, 1957.

________ "The Psychoanalytic Psychology of Imagination," *J. Amer. Psychoanal. Assoc.*, Vol. 8, pp. 252-269, 1960.

Bergler, E. "On the Resistence Situation: The Patient Is Silent," *Psychoanal. Rev.*, Vol. 25, p. 170, 1938.

Berndt, C. H., "Role of Native Doctors in Aboriginal Australia," In A. Kiev, ed., *Magic, Faith and Healing*. New York: Free Press, 1964.

Brazelton, T. B., "Crying in Infancy," *Pediatrics*, Vol. 29, p. 579, 1962.

Cohen, M. "Counter-Transference and Anxiety," *Psychiatry*, Vol. 15, pp. 231-243, 1952.

Colby, K. *A Primer for Psychotherapists*. New York: Ronald, 1951.

Deutsch, H. *The Psychology of Women*, 2 Vols. New York: Grune & Stratton, 1944, 1945.

Dunbar, F. *Emotions and Bodily Changes*. New York: Columbia University Press, 1954.

Enelow, A. J. "The Silent Patient," *Psychiatry*, Vol. 23, p. 153, 1960.

Ferenczi, S. "The Elasticity of Psychoanalytic Technique," in *Final Contributions to the Problems and Methods of Psycho-Analysis*. New York: Basic Books, 1955, pp. 87-101.

________ *Further Contributions to the Theory and Technique of Psycho-Analysis*. New York: Basic Books, 1953.

Ferreira, A. J. "The Intimacy Need in Psychotherapy," presented at the Vth International Congress of Psychotherapy, Vienna, 1961.

———. "Lonliness and Psychopathology," *Amer. J. of Psychoanal.*, Vol 22, p. 201, 1962.

———. "Psychotherapy with Severely Regressed Schizophrenics," *Psychiat. Quart.*, Vol. 33, p. 664, 1959.

Fliess, R. "Countertransference and Counter Identification," *J. Amer. Psychoanal. Assoc.*, Vol. 1, pp. 268-284, 1953.

———. "Silence and Verbalization: A Supplement to the Theory of the 'Analytic Rule,'" *Int. J. Psychoanal.*, Vol. 30, p. 21, 1949.

Foxe, A. N. "The Therapeutic Effect of Crying," *Medical Record*, Vol. 153, p. 167, 1941.

France, A. *The Wicker Work Woman, A Chronicle of Our Times*, M. P. Willcocks, trans., New York: Dodd, Mead, 1923.

Freud, S. *Complete Psychological Works of Sigmund Freud, Standard Edition*, James Strachey, trans. London: Hogarth, See esp. "Analysis Terminable and Unterminable," Vol. 23; "The Dynamics of Transference," Vol. 12; "The Ego and the Id," Vol. 19; "Female Sexuality," Vol. 21; "Fragment of an Analysis of a Case of Hysteria," Vol. 7; "Freud's Psychoanalytic Procedure," Vol. 7; "Further Recommendations in the Technique of Psycho-Analysis: Recollections, Repetition and Working Through," Vol. 2; "Group Psychology and the Analysis of the Ego," Vol. 18; "Inhibitions, Symptoms and Anxiety," Vol. ; "Interpretation of Dreams," Vol. 5; New Introductory Lectures on Psycho-Analysis,: Vol. 22; "Observations on Transference Love," Vol. 2; "On Narcissism," Vol. 4; "The Question of Lay Analysis," Vol. 20; "Recommendations to Physicians Practicing Psycho-Analysis," Vol. 12; "The Theme of Three Caskets, Vol. 4; "Totem and Taboo," Vol. 13; "Transformation of the Instincts," Vol. 2.

Fromm-Reichman, F. *Principles of Intensive Psychotherapy*. Chicago: University of Chicago Press, 1950.

Gill, M. M., R. Newman, F. C. Redlich. *The Initial Interview in Psychiatric Practice*; New York: International Universities Press, 1954.

Glover, E. *The Technique of Psycho-Analysis*, New York: International Universities Press, 1955.

Greenacre, P. "General Problems of Acting Out," in *Trauma, Growth and Personality*, New York: W. W. Norton, 1952, pp. 224-236.

———. "Pathological Weeping, *Psychoanalytic Quarterly*, Vol. 24, p. 62, 1945.

———. "The Role of Transference Practice Considerations in Relation to Psychoanalytic Theory," *J. Amer. Psychoanal. Assoc.*, Vol. 2, pp. 671-684, 1954.

Greene, A. B. *The Philosophy of Science*. New York: Richard R. Smith, 1940.

Greenson, R. R. "Empathy and Its Vicissitudes," *Int. J. of Psychoanal.*, Vol. 41, pp. 418-424, 1960.

———. "The Mother Tongue and the Mother," *Int. J. Psychoanal.*, Vol. 31, pp. 18-23, 1950.

———. "On the Silence and Sounds of the Analytic Hour," *J. Amer. Psychoanal. Assoc.*, Vol. 9, p. 79, 1961.

———. "The Working Alleavce and the Transference Neuroses," *Psychoanal. Quart.*, Vol. 34, pp. 155-181, 1965.

Gremm, K. L. J. *Uber Schenkennd Geben*. Berlin: Preussusche Academie der Wissenschaften, October 26, 1848.
Hartmann, H. "Notes on the Theory of Sublimation," in *Essays on Ego Psychology*, New York: International Universities Press, 1964, pp. 215-250.
Jones, E. "The Early Development of Female Sexuality," and "Introduction" in *Papers on Psychoanalysis*. Baltimore: William & Wilkens, 1948.
________. *Life and Work of Sigmund Freud*, Vols. I, II, III. New York: Basic Books, 1955.
Kaplan, B., and P. Johnson. "The Social Meaning of Navajo Psychopathology and Psychotherapy," in A. Kiev, ed., *Magic, Faith and Healing*. New York: Free Press, 1964.
Kardener, A. *The Individual and His Society*. New York: Columbia University Press, 1955.
Kelman, H. "Communing and Relating," *Amer. J. Psychother.*, Vol. 14, p. 70, 1960.
Klein, M. *Contributions of Psycho-Analysis*. London: Hogarth,
________. "Notes on Some Schizoid Mechanisms," *Int. J. Psycho-Anal.*, Vol. 27.
________. *Psychoanalysis of Children*. London: Hogarth.
Klein, M., and J. Riviere. *Love, Hate and Reparation*. London: Hogarth, 1937.
Kris, E. "Ego Psychology and Interpretation in Psychoanalytic Therapy," in *Psychoanal. Quart.*, Vol. 20, p. 18, 1951.
________. "On Preconsciousmental Processes," in *Psychoanalytic Exploration*, in Art. New York: International Universities Press, 1952.
LaCombe, P. A. "A Special Mechanism of Pathological Weeping," *Psychoanalytic Quarterly*, Vol. 27, p. 246, 1958.
LaRochefoucauld, F. *The Maxims of LaRochefoucauld*, L. Kronemberger, trans. New York: Random House, 1959.
Levy, L. "Silence in the Analytic Session," *Int. J. Psycho-Anal.*, Vol. 39, p. 50, 1958.
Lewinsky, H. "Pathological Generosity," *Int. J. Psycho-Anal.*, Vol. 32, p. 185, 1951.
Lief, H. T. "Silence as Intervention in Psycho-Therapy," *Amer. J. Psychoanal.*, Vol. 22, p. 80, 1962.
Lindemann, E. "Symptomatology and Management of Acute Grief," *Amer. J. Psychiat.*, Vol. 101, p. 140, 1944.
Little, M. "Transference in Borderline States," *Int. J. Psychoanal.*, Vol. 47, p. 4, 1966.
Loewald, H. W. "On the Therapeutic Action of Psycho-Analysis," *Int. J. Psychoanal.*, Vol. 41, pp. 16-33, 1960.
Loewenstein, R. M. "Some Remarks on the Role of Speech in Psycho-Analytic Technique," *Int. J. Psychoanal.*, Vol. 37, pp. 460-468, 1956.
Lorand, S. *Technique of Psychoanalytic Therapy*. New York: International Universities Press, 1946.
Lowen, A. *The Betrayal of the Body*, New York: Macmillan, 1966.
Marmor, J. "The Feeling of Superiority: An Occupational Hazard in Practice of Psychotherapy," *Amer. J. Psychiat.*, Vol. 110 (Nov.), p. 370, 1953.
Masserman, J. "Humanitarian Psychiatry," *Bull. N. Y. Acad. Med.*, Vol. 39, No. 8, 1963.
Mauss, M. *Gifts–Forms and Functions of Exchange in Archaic Societies*. London: Cohen & West, 1954.

McCartney, J. "Overt Transference," *J. Sex Research*, Vol. 2, No. 3, 1966.
Menninger, K. *Theory of Psychoanalytic Technique*, New York: Basic Books, 1958.
Meerloo, J. A. M. "Free Association, Silence and the Multiple Function of the Speech," *Psychiat. Quart.*, Vol. 26, p. 21, 1952.
_______. "Santa Claus and the Psychology of Giving," *Amer. Practitioner*, Vols. 11-12, pp. 1031-1035, 1960.
Money-Kyrles, R. *The Meaning of Sacrifice*. London: Hogarth, 1929.
Montagu, A. "National Selection and the Origin and Evolution of Weeping in Man," *Science*, Vol. 130, p. 1572, 1959.
Murphy, J. M. "Psychotherapeutic Aspects of Shamanism on St. Lawrence Island, Alaska," in A. Kiev, ed., *Magic, Faith and Healing*. New York: Free Press, 1964.
Nacht S. "Curative Factors in Psychoanalysis," *Int. J. of Psychoanal.*, Vol. 43, 1962.
_______. "Variations in Technique," *Int. J. Psychoanal.*, Vol. 39, 1958.
Nunberg, H. "The Will to Recover," in *Practice and Theory of Psychoanalysis*. New York: International Universities Press, 1955.
Perls, F. S., R. F. Hefferline, P. Goodman, *Gestalt Therapy*. New York: Dell, 1965.
Reik, T. *Listening with the Third Ear*. New York: Farrar, Strauss, 1948.
Rosen, U. H. "Some Aspects of the Role of Imagination in the Analytic Process," *J. Amer. Psychoanal. Assoc*. Vol. 8, pp. 229-251, 1960.
Rosenfeld, H. "Notes on the Psycho-Analysis of the Super Ego Conflict of the Acute Schizophrenic Patient," *Int. J. Psychoanal.*, Vol. 33, 1952.
Ruesch, J. and W. Kees. *Non-Verbal Communication*. Berkeley: University of California Press, 1959.
Ruitenbeek, Hendrik M., *Freud As We Knew Him*, Detroit, Wayne State University Press, 1973.
Rycroft, C. "The Nature and Function of the Analyst's Communication to the Patient," *Int. J. Psychoanal*, Vol. 37, pp. 469-472, 1956.
Schafer, R. "Generative Empathy in the Treatment Situation," *Psychoanalytic Quart.* Vol. 28, pp. 342-373, 1959.
Searles, H. "Transference Psychoses in the Psychotherapy of Schizophrenia," in *Collected Papers on Schizophrenia*. New York: International Universities Press, 1965.
Sechehaye, N. A. *Symbolic Realization*, New York: International Universities Press, 1951.
Segal, H. "Some Aspects of the Analysis of a Schizophrenic," *Int. J. Psychoanal.* Vol. 31, 1956.
Selzer, M. "The Happy College Student Myth: Psychiatric Implications," *American Medical Association, Arch. Gen. Psychiatry and Neurology* Vol. 2, p. 131 (Feb.), 1960.
Sharpe, E. "Psycho-physical Problems Revealed in Language: An Examination of Metaphore," and "The Technique of Psychoanalysis," in *Collected Papers on Psychoanalysis*. London: Hogarth, 1950, pp. 109-122.
Simmel, E. "The 'Doctor-Game' Illness and the Profession of Medicine," *Int. J. of Psychoanal.*, Vol. 7, pp. 470-483, 1926.
Spitz, R. "Countertransference: Comments on Its Varying Role in the Analytic Situation," *J. Amer. Psychoanal. Assoc.*, Vol. 4, pp. 256-265, 1956.
Sterba, R. "The Dynamic of the Dissolution of the Transference Resistence," *Psychoanal. Quart.*, Vol. 9, pp. 363-379. 1940.

Szasz, T. S. "On the Experiences of the Analyst in the Psychoanalytic Situation: A Contribution to the Theory of Psychoanalytic Treatment," *J. Amer. Psychoanal. Assoc.* Vol. 4, pp. 197-223, 1956.

Versteeg-Solleveld, C. M. "De Silence," *Folia Psychiatry*, Vol. 55, p. 150, 1952.

Veitt, I. *Hysteria: The History of a Disease*. Chicago: University of Chicago Press, 1965.

Weigert, E. "Lonliness and Trust–Basic Features of Human Existence," *Psychiatry*, Vol. 23, p. 121, 1960.

Weisman, A. D. "Silence and Psychotherapy," *Psychiatry*, Vol. 18, p. 241, 1955.

Winnicott, D. W. "Hate in the Counter Transference," *Int. J. Psychoanal.*, Vol. 30, pp. 69-74, 1949.

________. Metta Psychological and Chemical Aspects of Regression within the Psycho-Analytic Setup," in *Collected Papers*. New York: Basic Books, pp. 278-294, 1958.

Wolberg, L. R. *The Technique of Psycho-therapy*. New York: Grune & Stratton, 1954.

Wolstein, B. *Counter Transference.* New York: Grune & Stratton, 1959.

Zeligs, M. A. "The Psychology of Science," *J. Amer. Psychoanal. Assoc.*, Vol. 9, p. 7, 1961.

Zetzel, E. "Current Concepts of Transference," *Int. J. Psychoanal.*, Vol. 37, pp. 369-376, 1956.

Index